Developmental Psychobiology

Review of Psychiatry Series
John M. Oldham, M.D., M.S.
Michelle B. Riba, M.D., M.S.
Series Editors

Developmental Psychobiology

EDITED BY

B.J. Casey, Ph.D.

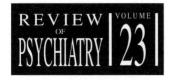

REVIEW OF PSYCHIATRY | VOLUME 23

No. 4

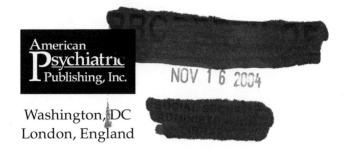

American Psychiatric Publishing, Inc.

Washington, DC
London, England

Copyright © 2004 American Psychiatric Publishing, Inc.
ALL RIGHTS RESERVED

Manufactured in the United States of America on acid-free paper
08 07 06 05 04   5 4 3 2 1
First Edition

Typeset in Adobe's Palatino

American Psychiatric Publishing, Inc.
1000 Wilson Boulevard
Arlington, VA 22209-3901
www.appi.org

The correct citation for this book is
   Casey BJ (editor): *Developmental Psychobiology* (Review of Psychiatry Series, Volume 23; Oldham JM and Riba MB, series editors). Washington, DC, American Psychiatric Publishing, 2004

Library of Congress Cataloging-in-Publication Data
Developmental psychobiology / edited by B.J. Casey.
       p. ; cm. — (Review of psychiatry ; v. 23, no. 4)
   Includes bibliographical references and index.
   ISBN 1-58562-176-5 (alk. paper)
      1. Biological child psychiatry. 2. Developmental psychobiology. I. Casey, B.J., 1960– II. Review of psychiatry series ; v. 23, 4.
   [DNLM: 1. Biological Psychiatry. 2. Developmental Biology. 3. Child Psychiatry. WM 102 D489 2004]
   RJ486.5.D485 2004
   618.92'89–dc22

                                                                    200307891

British Library Cataloguing in Publication Data
A CIP record is available from the British Library.

Contents

Contributors

B.J. Casey, Ph.D.
Director, Sackler Institute for Developmental Psychobiology, Weill Medical College of Cornell University, New York, New York

Susan L. Erickson, Ph.D.
Postdoctoral Fellow, Department of Neurobiology, University of Pittsburgh, Pittsburgh, Pennsylvania

Kathy A. Gallardo, M.D., Ph.D.
Psychiatry Resident, Department of Psychiatry, Yale University, New Haven, Connecticut

Myron A. Hofer, M.D.
Sackler Institute Professor of Developmental Psychobiology, Department of Psychiatry, Columbia University and New York State Psychiatric Institute, New York, New York

James F. Leckman, M.D.
Nelson Harris Professor and Director of Research, Child Study Center and the Departments of Pediatrics, Psychiatry, and Psychology, Yale University, New Haven, Connecticut

David A. Lewis, M.D.
Professor, Department of Psychiatry, University of Pittsburgh, Pittsburgh, Pennsylvania

Bruce D. McCandliss, Ph.D.
Assistant Professor of Psychology in Psychiatry, Sackler Institute for Developmental Psychobiology, Weill Medical College of Cornell University, New York, New York

Charles A. Nelson, Ph.D.
Distinguished McKnight University Professor of Child Psychology, Pediatrics, and Neuroscience; Nancy M. and John E. Lindahl Professor for Excellence in Teaching and Learning, Institute of Child Development, Center for Cognitive Sciences, Center for Neurobehavioral Development, University of Minnesota, Minneapolis, Minnesota

John M. Oldham, M.D., M.S.
Professor and Chair, Department of Psychiatry and Behavioral Sciences, Medical University of South Carolina, Charleston, South Carolina

Michelle B. Riba, M.D., M.S.
Clinical Professor and Associate Chair for Education and Academic Affairs, Department of Psychiatry, University of Michigan Medical School, Ann Arbor, Michigan

Lisa S. Scott, B.S.
Doctoral Candidate, Institute of Child Development, Center for Cognitive Sciences, Center for Neurobehavioral Development, University of Minnesota, Minneapolis, Minnesota

James E. Swain, M.D., Ph.D.
Postdoctoral Associate, Child Study Center, Yale University, New Haven, Connecticut

Michael Wolmetz, B.S.
Research Aide, Sackler Institute for Developmental Psychobiology, Weill Medical College of Cornell University, New York, New York

Introduction to the Review of Psychiatry Series

John M. Oldham, M.D., M.S.
Michelle B. Riba, M.D., M.S., Series Editors

2004 REVIEW OF PSYCHIATRY SERIES TITLES

- *Developmental Psychobiology*
  EDITED BY B.J. CASEY, PH.D.
- *Neuropsychiatric Assessment*
  EDITED BY STUART C. YUDOFSKY, M.D., AND H. FLORENCE KIM, M.D.
- *Brain Stimulation in Psychiatric Treatment*
  EDITED BY SARAH H. LISANBY, M.D.
- *Cognitive-Behavior Therapy*
  EDITED BY JESSE H. WRIGHT, M.D., PH.D.

Throughout the country, media coverage is responding to increased popular demand for information about the brain—what it does, how it works, and what to expect of it throughout the life cycle. For example, in a special issue of *Scientific American* called "Better Brains: How Neuroscience Will Enhance You," in September 2003, leading researchers summarized exciting new frontiers in psychiatry, including neuroplasticity, new diagnostic technology, new drug development informed by knowledge about gene sequences and molecular configurations, new directions in stress management guided by increased understanding of the effects of stress on the brain, and brain stimulation techniques related to the revolutionary recognition that neurogenesis can occur in the adult brain. This special issue illustrates the enormous excitement about developments in brain science.

In our scientific journals, there is an explosion of information about neuroscience and about the bidirectional nature of brain and behavior. The matter was previously debated as if one had to choose between two camps (mind versus brain), but a rapidly developing new paradigm is replacing this former dichotomy—that the brain influences behavior, and that the mind (ideas, emotions, hopes, aspirations, anxieties, fears, and the wide realm of real and perceived environmental experience) influences the brain. The term *neuropsychiatry* has served as successor to the former term *organic psychiatry* and is contrasted with notions of psychodynamics, such as the concept of unconsciously motivated behavior. As our field evolves and matures, we are developing a new language for meaningful but imperfectly understood earlier concepts. *Subliminal cues* and *indirect memory* are among the terms of our new language, but the emerging understanding that experience itself can activate genes and stimulate protein synthesis, cellular growth, and neurogenesis is a groundbreaking new synthesis of concepts that previously seemed incompatible. Among the remarkable conclusions that these new findings suggest is that psychotherapy can be construed as a biological treatment, in the sense that it has the potential to alter the cellular microanatomy of the brain.

In the context of this rapidly changing scientific and clinical landscape, we selected for the 2004 Review of Psychiatry four broad areas of attention: 1) research findings in developmental psychobiology, 2) current recommendations for neuropsychiatric assessment of patients, 3) new treatments in the form of brain stimulation techniques, and 4) the application of cognitive-behavior therapy as a component of treatment of patients with severely disabling psychiatric disorders.

Perhaps the logical starting place in the 2004 series is *Developmental Psychobiology*, edited by B.J. Casey. Derived from research that uses animal models and studies of early human development, this work summarizes the profound impact of early environmental events. Following a comprehensive overview of the field by Casey, elegant studies of the developmental psychobiology of attachment are presented by Hofer, one of the pioneers in this work. Specific areas of research are then described in detail: the developmental neurobiology of an early maturational task called face processing (Scott and Nelson); findings in the developmental psychobiology of reading disability (McCandliss and Wolmetz); current thinking about the central relevance of early development in the disabling condition Gilles de la Tourette's syndrome (Gallardo, Swain, and Leckman); and the early development of the prefrontal cortex and the implications of these findings in adult-onset schizophrenia (Erickson and Lewis).

Stuart C. Yudofsky and H. Florence Kim, the editors of *Neuropsychiatric Assessment,* have gathered together experts to bring us up to date on the current practice of neuropsychiatric physical diagnosis (Ovsiew); the importance of the neuropsychological examination of psychiatric patients (Getz and Lovell); and the use of electrophysiological testing (Boutros and Struve) and neuropsychiatric laboratory testing (Kim and Yudofsky) in clinical practice. Any focus on neuropsychiatry today must include information about developments in brain imaging; here the clinical usefulness of selected neuroimaging techniques for specific psychiatric disorders is reviewed by Nordahl and Salo.

A particularly interesting area of clinical research, and one with promising potential to provide new treatment techniques, is that of stimulating the brain. The long-known phenomenon of "magnetism" has emerged in a fascinating new incarnation, referred to in its central nervous system applications as transcranial magnetic stimulation (TMS). Sarah H. Lisanby edited *Brain Stimulation in Psychiatric Treatment,* in which TMS is described in connection with its possible use in depression (Schlaepfer and Kosel) and in schizophrenia and other disorders (Hoffman). New applications in psychiatry of deep brain stimulation, a technique showing great promise in Parkinson's disease and other neurological conditions, are reviewed (Greenberg), and the current state of knowledge about magnetic seizure therapy (Lisanby) and vagal nerve stimulation (Sackeim) is presented. All of these roads of investigation have the potential to lead to new, perhaps more effective treatments for our patients.

Finally, in *Cognitive-Behavior Therapy,* edited by Jesse H. Wright, the broadening scope of cognitive therapy is considered with regard to schizophrenia (Scott, Kingdon, and Turkington), bipolar disorder (Basco, McDonald, Merlock, and Rush), medical patients (Sensky), and children and adolescents (Albano, Krain, Podniesinksi, and Ditkowsky). Technological advances in the form of computer-assisted cognitive behavior therapy are presented as well (Wright).

All in all, in our view the selected topics for 2004 represent a rich sampling of the amazing developments taking place in brain science and psychiatric evaluation and treatment. We believe that we have put together an equally relevant menu for 2005, when the Review of Psychiatry Series will include volumes on psychiatric genetics (Kenneth Kendler, editor); sleep disorders and psychiatry (Daniel Buysse, editor); pregnancy and postpartum depression (Lee Cohen, editor); and bipolar disorder (Terence Ketter, Charles Bowden, and Joseph Calabrese, editors).

Introduction

B.J. Casey, Ph.D.

Developmental psychobiology is a multidisciplinary field, and any discipline that impinges on or informs us about development is thus important to the field of developmental psychobiology. The chapters in this volume reflect a broad sampling of work that addresses three fundamental topics on understanding typical and atypical development. These topics are particularly relevant to biological and child psychiatry, and the three fundamental topics listed below are discussed in greater detail later in this Introduction to provide essential background information for subsequent chapters:

1. **The importance of both plasticity and stability in the development of behavioral and neural systems.** The development and maturation of the organism is a careful balance between certain amounts of *plasticity* as well as *stability*. Too much plasticity can hinder long-term forms of learning, whereas a system that is too stable can be devastating to the normal functioning of the organism, particularly in the case where atypical behaviors and neural representations have formed. The interplay of plasticity and stability is addressed by Hofer in Chapter 1, which contains a review of the literature on early attachment.

2. **Establishment of typical and atypical developmental progressions in systems.** Understanding the normal development of behavioral and neural systems is critical to interpreting and investigating atypical development. A number of behaviors may be completely appropriate at one age but inappropriate at another age. Clinical disorders may reflect exaggerated and/or residual behaviors and neural processes that do not necessarily diminish or change with maturity. These behaviors are typically examined in terms of either developmental delays or deficiencies. Understanding normal progressions in behavioral and

neural systems will have a significant impact in determining the biological substrates of clinical disorders and targeting effective treatments and interventions. This topic is perhaps best illustrated in the chapter by Gallardo, Swain, and Leckman on Tourette's syndrome (Chapter 4) and Erickson and Lewis on schizophrenia (Chapter 5).

3. **The impact of methodological advances on imaging and genetics in understanding typical and atypical behavioral and neural development.** This volume addresses how developments in noninvasive tools for looking into the developing, behaving human brain have helped to inform or constrain our understanding of typical and atypical development. Historically, biological psychiatry has been based on work stemming from psychopharmacological studies, but now together with imaging and genetic techniques one can further characterize the biological mechanisms underlying a disorder. Aspects of this topic are covered across all five chapters of this volume, but Scott and Nelson's review of the development of face processing (Chapter 2) and McCandliss and Wolmetz's review of the development of word reading (Chapter 3) provide elegant examples of the impact of imaging on our understanding of typical and atypical development in these areas.

The chapters in this volume emphasize the role of plasticity and stability in learning, the typical and atypical progressions of development, and the methods for studying such learning and development. These elements underscore the importance of viewing the organism in terms of dynamically changing behavioral and neural processes. This multifaceted approach is especially important for understanding clinical disorders that show a) atypical progressions in behavior, such as episodic changes (waxing and waning of symptoms) in Tourette's syndrome and obsessive-compulsive disorder; or b) the discontinuation or lack of progression in adaptive behaviors, such as eye contact and gaze in autism, word reading in dyslexia, and aspects of working memory in schizophrenia.

Balancing Plasticity and Stability During Development

Why is learning enhanced in the developing organism? How does experience shape behavior and how does the nature of these experiences result in stable, less plastic behavioral and neural representations? These questions are perhaps some of the most interesting in developmental psychobiology because they suggest critical or sensitive periods of behavioral and neural development during which the system may be primed for, or more sensitive to, a particular experience.

Characteristics of Developmental Learning

Developmental learning refers to enhanced effects of experiences in the immature system relative to the mature system. Sensitive and critical periods are a form of developmental learning that differ from mature learning in the speed, quantity, and quality of learning. A *sensitive period* may be defined as a stage of development when the brain is *experience expectant,* or especially sensitive to modification by experience. Learning in the sensitive period differs from learning in the critical period. In the *critical period* of learning, experience was thought to be essential for normal brain development *(experience dependent)* and without the experience, the cognitive and neural systems were assumed not to develop appropriately. Critical periods then suggest an irreversible and permanent change, whereas sensitive periods suggest greater flexibility in the system with the potential to be reversible with later appropriate experiences or intervention. Thus sensitive periods offer more plasticity than critical periods and appear to more accurately reflect human learning and development.

Plasticity in developmental learning refers to the capacity for adjustment or modification in the neural and behavioral systems of the organism. Basically some degree of adaptive plasticity continues throughout the life span of an animal, but this plasticity appears greatest in the developing organism. Critical periods, however, result in learning that has little ability for later change.

The organism must be in a state of biological readiness to benefit from new experiences. So the opening of a sensitive period of behavioral development is dependent on neuronal maturation. After a sensitive period of development is presumably closed, experiences encountered will have little effect on the organism. Sensitive periods are thought to "end" once the individual has received adequate experience and a neural pathway is "irreversibly" committed to a particular pattern of neuronal connectivity. The neural basis for such irreversibility has not been established. Multiple processes may underlie this change. There is speculation that synaptic efficacy such as long-term potentiation and depression as well as growth proteins responsible for large-scale axonal growth are altered permanently by adequate experience, but the relative plasticity shown in even mature systems suggests that other mechanisms may be involved.

The development and maturation of the organism is a careful balance between plasticity and stability (see Figure 1). Too much plasticity could hinder long-term learning, whereas too much stability could result in the early formation of aberrant behavioral or neural representations. Chapter 1 focuses on early attachment, discussing the bond, the response to separation, and the long-term effects of the early relationship.

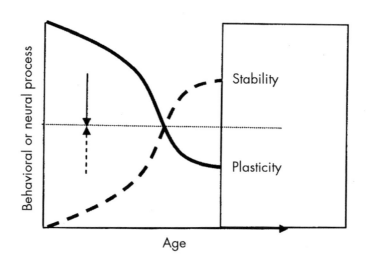

Figure 1. Illustration of the relation between plasticity and stability in the development of behavioral and neural representations.

In Chapter 1, Hofer includes a review of the intriguing human and animal work on the infant's early recognition of his or her own mother. For example, the newborn in the first few hours of birth will prefer native language over another, female voices over male, and mother's voice reading over another mother's (DeCasper and Fifer 1980; Fifer and Moon 1995). Newborns appear to prefer stimuli similar to ones with which they have had repeated, early experience. Thus experiences even during fetal development determine later long-term behavioral preferences.

Striking cross-species similarities are observed in such preferences as shown in rat pups' preferences to their own dam's amniotic fluid relative to another dam's (Hepper 1987). Experience-based learning of contingent events in the newborn rat pup have been shown (Sullivan et al. 1986) using a novel odor and simulated licking of the pup (stroking with soft brush). This manipulation resulted in the rat pup approaching and remaining close to the odor. Such stimulation ceased to induce preferences after the first postnatal week and by the second week began to induce avoidance responses. These results define a sensitive period of enhanced learning and plasticity, resulting in the formation of positive associations that were reinforced by tactile simulation as the odor came to elicit behaviors similar to those during interaction with the dam.

This rapid learning process resembles that of filial imprinting (the rapid ability to distinguish the parent from others) in geese as described by Konrad Lorenz. Yet Hofer poignantly suggests that such rapid learning reminds us of the clinical observation that long-lasting attachments can occur in children even with abusive parents. Perhaps this observation alone is sufficient to underscore the importance of both plasticity and stability in typical and atypical development. A system that is too stable, particularly in the case of early attachment, can be devastating to the normal functioning of the organism in the cases of neglect and abuse that affect the general well-being and health of the organism long term (McEwen 2003).

Mechanisms Underlying Developmental Learning

Why do there appear to be sensitive periods in development, during which learning, whether aberrant or typical, is enhanced?

Computational models, specifically neural network simulations, have been employed to investigate potential mechanisms for sensitive periods (e.g., Ellis and Lambon Ralph 2000; Zevin and Seidenberg 2002). These models allow researchers to exercise complete control over simulated learning systems and their environments, to help identify factors contributing to enhanced learning during particular points in development.

Neural network simulations have been used to investigate the possibility that sensitive periods arise because knowledge becomes entrenched as a system learns, making system alterations more difficult with subsequent learning (Munakata et al. (in press). Such simulations have demonstrated how entrenchment can arise as units and connections become committed and as unused connections are pruned (Ellis and Lambon Ralph 2000; Zevin and Seidenberg 2002). As a result, stimuli that are encountered early are learned more robustly than stimuli encountered later.

Entrenchment or stability can occur due to counterproductive learning, whereby incorrect responses are strengthened. Neural network simulations have demonstrated how such processes could lead to sensitive periods in phoneme discrimination (McClelland et al. 1999). Specifically, an infant (or network) may start with an auditory perceptual system that responds differentially to sounds in the environment, and strengthens these responses with experience. After neurons become recruited to represent sounds in one language environment, it can be difficult for the system to represent sounds of a different language. For example, a learner in a Japanese language environment will experience a sound that is a blend of the English /r/ and /l/ sounds. This sound will activate relevant neurons, and learning will lead to a strengthening of this response. If later faced with an English /r/ or /l/, the existing representation of the single blended sound will be activated in this system. Learning will again tend to strengthen this response, but in this case the learning will be counterproductive, strengthening the tendency to hear the English /r/ and /l/ sounds as the single blended sound. The interaction of these learning processes and environmental inputs can thus lead to sensitive periods for learning phonemes, as demonstrated by the simulations.

An example of developmental learning is described by Scott and Nelson (Chapter 2) in their review of the face processing literature. They characterize face processing as an experience-expectant process, with a "period of opportunity," for the development of this perceptual ability, when visual face information present in the environment molds the specificity of this system. McCandliss and Wolmetz (Chapter 3) describe a similar form of developmental learning in the context of word reading. From the developmental psychobiology perspective, acquisition of literacy represents a unique domain involving experience-driven interactions between language and visual systems during relatively different stages of development. In their chapter they consider how the brain systems that support these processes change over the course of the acquisition of reading skill, how individual differences in these brain mechanisms impact course of reading development (i.e., phonological deficits and reading disabilities), and how cognitive interventions impact the brain systems involved.

Typical and Atypical Developmental Progressions

Behavioral change over the course of development is no doubt a reflection of complex changes and interactions in experiences, genes, and hormones. Defining developmental trajectories in behavior and neural representations is therefore critical in the characterization of how they go awry in developmental disabilities (see Figure 2).

Biological changes can occur in the absence of specific experience or stimulation. For example, during early development, an overproduction of synapses is followed by a subsequent decline in number of synapses. Presumably experience selects which of these synapses survive. However, if we expose the developing organism to experiences earlier than expected by bringing the animal into the world prematurely or prevent experiences by blocking sensory input with visual occlusion, an overproduction of synapses and subsequent decline still occur (Bourgeois et al. 1989). Thus the developmental trajectory in number of synapses appears to be genet-

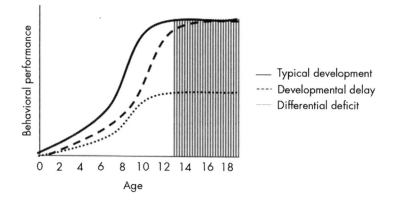

Figure 2. Model of developmental progressions of typical and atypical (delayed, deficient) behavioral and neural processes.

ically preprogrammed providing a scaffold upon which further experiences can build. It would be an oversimplification to try to dissociate genetic processes (nature) from experience-based ones (nurture) as we know that experiences can profoundly affect gene expression.

Some of the more interesting phenomena in development behave nonlinearly rather than linearly. This type of developmental trend suggests different mechanisms may come to support a behavior if that behavior is present, then absent, and subsequently returns over time. In this context, it is more difficult to think of the immature system as a little adult as qualitative shifts in development are inconsistent with gradual continuous change.

Phenomena that can be accounted for by linear increases or decreases suggest quantitative refinement in a fairly intact system. In this context, theorists often think of the immature system as a little adult with only minor quantitative changes needed to reach the mature state. A number of examples where steady growth or refinement of an intact system have been suggested to account for developmental change. For example, linear changes in speed of processing in children's behavioral responses have been suggested to be due to changes in myelination of axons. Myelin growth increases efficiency in neuronal conduction by as much as 50% and thus seems like a plausible explanation even though the rate and thickness of myelin cannot be measured precisely in vivo and related directly to behavioral change quantitatively. Other processes could also explain some of the change (e.g., synaptic pruning, vasculature changes, dendritic branching). Such claims of causality between coincidental changes in brain and behavioral development are commonly reported but rarely empirically grounded.

Gallardo, Swain, and Leckman in their chapter on Tourette's syndrome provide an example of the importance in characterizing developmental progressions and changes in tic disorders. Such an approach allows one to ask why tics appear when they do or why motor tics appear before vocal tics. Why do tics wax and wane? Why do they reach a worst-ever point in early adolescence, for a majority, and become even more severe in adulthood for an unlucky few? These questions suggest the importance of timing and behavioral progressions when evaluating the neural basis of this disorder.

Most of the neural evidence for Tourette's syndrome points to the involvement of cortico-striato-thalamo-cortical circuits being crucial for the development of habits, tics, and stereotypies, yet the precise mechanisms remain in question. Given the developmental progressions of this disorder, mapping behavioral changes with known development of this circuitry may be the most effective approach to understanding the disorder. Developmental shifts in dopamine-related modulation of this circuitry have been implicated in tic severity (Wolf et al. 1996), and pediatric cases of streptococcal-infection–related post-infectious autoimmune mechanisms have been implicated in the waxing and waning of symptoms (Swedo et al. 1998). Thus, understanding the timing and maturation of cortico-striato-thalamo-cortical circuitry may shed light on critical windows of vulnerability in the development and timing of tics.

Another example of developmental progressions in the behavioral and neural processes underlying a disorder is described by Erickson and Lewis (Chapter 5) in their review of schizophrenia. Postnatal developmental changes that occur in the circuitry of the dorsolateral prefrontal cortex appear to underlie maturation of working memory, a function disrupted in schizophrenia.

Attempts to produce a unifying concept of the etiology of schizophrenia have posited that biological mechanisms with origins in developmental processes occur before the onset of clinical symptoms. Although agreement has not yet been achieved regarding the specific causal factors and the time frame during which these mechanisms may act, the neurodevelopmental nature of schizophrenia appears to be a particularly attractive model. These postnatal developmental changes may inform our understanding of the disturbances of this circuitry and their function in schizophrenia.

Impact of Methodological Advances on the Field

Developments in the human genome project and in magnetic resonance imaging (MRI) methods provide us with the opportunity to more directly examine the effects of early experience on gene expression and plasticity in the developing human brain. These methods also offer new directions in biological psychiatry. We are in an explosive era of methodological development that has opened new doors for examining the developing human brain in vivo. Functional neuroimaging is providing new insights into the dynamics of neural circuits involved in cognitive and emotional development and genomic research is producing an abundance of new target molecules for the treatment of developmental disorders. With this progress, new efforts are under way to unify the understanding of functional brain anatomy with physiological, cellular, and molecular processes that influence behavior. For example, Fan et al. (2003) and others (Egan et al. 2001) have shown how genetic variants can impact the activity of brain regions implicated in well-defined behaviors with combined imaging and genetic studies (see Figure 3). Such approaches are only beginning to be used with developmental and clinical populations. A unified understanding of mechanisms involved in cognitive and emotional development may open up new avenues for therapeutic intervention for clinical populations at the pharmacological, genetic, and behavioral levels.

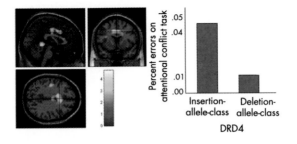

Figure 3. Allelic variation in the dopamine receptor (DRD4) gene and functional magnetic resonance imaging–based brain activity.

Greater brain activity among subjects who were grouped according to genotype at the DRD4 insertion class ($n=6$) in comparison with deletion class ($n=10$). The *color bar* represents the level of t value. The graph shows the error rate during an attentional conflict task for each genetic group. More errors relate to greater cingulate activity for the DRD4 insertion class.

Source. Adapted from Fan et al. 2003.

Recent progress in the field of developmental psychobiology is most evident in the growing number of biological studies on human brain development. Perhaps the most obvious examples are those involving noninvasive MRI. Although it is true that progress in imaging methods offers a new window into the developing, behaving, human brain (Casey 2002; Casey and de Haan 2002), other methods including animal and computational models, lesion studies, and genetics remain essential in constraining the interpretation of imaging data, informing theories of behavioral and brain development, and encouraging new interventions for atypically developing populations (Casey and Munakata 2002; Posner et al. 2001; Johnson 2001).

With noninvasive functional imaging methods, we can repeatedly and safely image the same subjects multiple times to track changes in cortical activation following practice or training. Such an approach may provide a more definitive test of whether developmental differences are maturation- or experience-based by assessing brain activity both before and following training. Karni et al. (1995) have shown rapid learning effects in primary motor areas in adults during motor sequence learning within a single session that increased over weeks of training. The activity in motor cortex became less diffuse and increased over time.

The example of initial diffuse cortical activity early in learning, followed by an increase in focal activity, parallels results from developmental functional MRI (fMRI) studies. These studies show diffuse activity in children relative to adolescents and adults, with adolescents showing the greatest focal activity during performance of behavioral tasks, even when performance is equated across age groups (Casey et al. 1997, 2002; Hertz-Pannier et al. 1997; Klingberg et al. 2001; Schlagger et al. 2002). These studies do not necessarily indicate that differences in brain activity between age groups is due to experience alone, because even without normal stimulation, changes in neuronal connections and synaptic pruning occur with development (Bourgeois et al. 1994). Rather, these findings highlight a possible approach for addressing the maturation versus experience question.

To determine whether the immature system engages in the same neural mechanisms as the mature one after extended practice, we could examine brain activity both before and following extended experience. These findings highlight the use of fMRI to trace learning-related changes in cortical areas and will no doubt be informative when investigating the impact of behavioral training and interventions for reading problems or other cognitive skill development as those described in the context of face processing (Chapter 2) and word reading (Chapter 3).

Conclusion

This volume on developmental psychobiology emphasizes the importance of examining developmental progressions and changes in typical and atypical behavioral and neural systems. Both plasticity and stability in the development of these systems are a critical part of these progressions. Clearly, imaging, computational modeling, and genetic techniques will continue to inform us about progressions in typically and atypically developing populations.

The work collected in this volume suggests that biological and child psychiatry is in a new era, moving from solely psychopharmacological investigations of biological substrates of disorders to a more unified understanding of mechanisms involved in cognitive and emotional disorders with the use of imaging and genetic methods. Such approaches may open new avenues for therapeutic intervention for clinical populations at the pharmacological, genetic, and behavioral levels.

References

Bourgeois JP, Jastreboff PJ, Rakic P: Synaptogenesis in visual cortex of normal and preterm monkeys: evidence for intrinsic regulation of synaptic overproduction. Proc Natl Acad Sci U S A 86:4297–4301, 1989

Bourgeois JP, Goldman-Rakic PS, Rakic P: Synaptogenesis in the prefrontal cortex of rhesus monkeys. Cereb Cortex 4:78–96, 1994

Casey BJ: Windows into the developing human brain. Science 296:1408–1409, 2002

Casey BJ, de Haan M: Imaging methods in developmental science. Developmental Science 5:265–267, 2002

Casey BJ, Munakata Y: Converging methods in developmental science: an introduction. Dev Psychobiol 40:197–199, 2002

Casey BJ, Trainor RJ, Orendi JL, et al: A developmental functional MRI study of prefrontal activation during performance of a go–no-go task. J Cogn Neurosci 9:835–847, 1997

Casey BJ, Thomas KM, Davidson MC, et al: Dissociating striatal and hippocampal function developmentally with a stimulus-response compatibility task. J Neurosci 22: 8647–8652, 2002

DeCasper AJ, Fifer WP: Of human bonding: newborns prefer their mothers' voices. Science 208:1174–1176, 1980

Egan MF, Goldberg TE, Kolachana BS, et al: Effect of COMT Val108/158 Met genotype on frontal lobe function and risk for schizophrenia. Proc Natl Acad Sci U S A 98:6917–6922, 2001

Ellis AW, Lambon Ralph MA: Age of acquisition effects in adult lexical processing reflect loss of plasticity in maturing systems: insights from connectionist networks. J Exp Psychol Learn Mem Cogn 26:1103–1123, 2000

Fan J, Fossella J, Sommer T, et al: Mapping the genetic variation of executive attention onto brain activity. Proc Natl Acad Sci U S A 100:7406–7411, 2003

Fifer WP, Moon CM: The effects of fetal experience with sound, in *Fetal Development: a Psychobiological Perspective*. Edited by Lecanuet J-P, Fifer WP, Krasnegor NA, et al. Lawrence Erlbaum Associates, Hillsdale, New Jersey, 1995, pp 351–368

Hepper PG: The amniotic fluid: an important priming role in kin recognition. Anim Behav 35:1343–46, 1987

Hertz-Pannier L, Gaillard WD, Mott SH, et al: Noninvasive assessment of language dominance in children and adolescents with functional MRI: a preliminary study. Neurology 48:1003–1012, 1997

Johnson MH: Functional brain development in humans. Nat Rev Neurosci 2:475–483, 2001

Karni A, Meyer G, Jezzard P, et al: Functional MRI evidence for adult motor cortex plasticity during motor skill learning. Nature 377:155–158, 1995

Klingberg T, Forssberg H, Westerberg H: Increased brain activity in frontal and parietal cortex underlies the development of visuospatial working memory capacity during childhood. J Cogn Neurosci 14:1–10, 2001

McClelland JL, Thomas AG, McCandliss BD, et al: Understanding failures of learning: Hebbian learning, competition for representational space, and some preliminary experimental data. Prog Brain Res 121:75–80, 1999

McEwen B: Early life influence on life-long patterns of behavior and health. Ment Retard Dev Disabil Res Rev 9:149–154, 2003

Munakata Y, Casey BJ, Diamond A: Developmental cognitive neuroscience: progress and potential. Trends Cogn Sci (in press)

Posner MI, Rothbart M, Farah M, et al: The developing human brain. Developmental Science 4:253–387, 2001

Schlaggar BL, Brown TT, Lugar HM, et al: Functional neuroanatomical differences between adults and school-age children in the processing of single words. Science 296:1476–1479, 2002

Sullivan RM, Hofer MA, Brake SC: Olfactory-guided orientation in neonatal rats is enhanced by a conditioned change in behavioral state. Dev Psychobiol 19:615–623, 1986

Swedo SE, Leonard HL, Garvey M, et al: Pediatric autoimmune neuropsychiatric disorders associated with streptococcal infections: clinical description of the first 50 cases. Am J Psychiatry 155:264–271, 1998

Wolf SS, Jones DW, Knable MB, et al: Tourette syndrome: prediction of phenotypic variation in monozygotic twins by caudate nucleus D2 receptor binding. Science 273:1225–1227, 1996

Zevin J, Seidenberg M: Age of acquisition effects in reading and other tasks. Journal of Memory and Language 47:1–29, 2002

Chapter 1

Developmental Psychobiology of Early Attachment

Myron A. Hofer, M.D.

In the last decade, there has been growing awareness of the magnitude of the problem of child maltreatment. According to the National Center for Child Abuse and Neglect, 1.5 million verified cases of child maltreatment are reported annually in the United States (Margolis and Gordis 2002). More than half of these involve neglect; the others are cases of physical, sexual, and emotional abuse. The long-term consequences of this public health menace to infants and children also have become evident in the number of studies showing an increased risk of depression, anxiety disorders, and posttraumatic stress disorder in adults with histories of early abuse as infants and children (reviewed in Heim and Nemeroff 2001).

The recent clinical data, and an awareness of new research findings coming from behavioral neuroscience laboratories

Research covered in this chapter was supported by The Sackler Institute for Developmental Psychobiology at Columbia University, a Research Scientist Award (5 K05 MH38632), and a Project Grant (5 R01 MH40430) from the National Institute of Mental Health.

Parts of this chapter were adapted from Hofer MA: "Origins of Attachment and Regulators of Development Within Social Interactions: From Animal to Human," in *Handbook of Brain and Behavior in Human Development*. Edited by Kalverboer AF, Gramsbergen A. Dordrecht, The Netherlands, Kluwer Academic Publishers, 2001. Copyright 2001 Kluwer Academic Publishers. Used with kind permission of Kluwer Academic Publishers.

studying early development of the parent–infant interaction, have stimulated increasing interest in early attachment among psychiatrists over the past decade. Historically, the place of the infantile attachment concept has been an uncertain one, not only in psychiatry but also in developmental psychobiology itself. John Bowlby was knighted by the Queen of England but disregarded by his psychoanalytic colleagues. His ideas did not fare much better among those studying the behavioral and biological processes of early development. I cannot recall using the word *attachment* in my research or hearing it from my colleagues in developmental psychobiology during my first 20 years in the field. The concept was too global and did not readily suggest research questions that would advance our understanding of its nature and how it functioned. Outside of psychoanalysis and developmental psychobiology, however, Bowlby's attachment theory (Bowlby 1969) inspired remarkable changes in the treatment of infants, young children, and their parents and gave rise to an enormous body of research by developmental psychologists based on Mary Ainsworth's (Bowlby's colleague and successor) research instrument known as "The Strange Situation."

Bowlby's great accomplishment was to dispel the misconception that existed among professionals in the first half of the twentieth century—that the only functions of the mother for the infant were to provide nutrition and protection. Too much time spent with the mother in trivial play, it was thought, would only serve to delay the development of independence and reason. But it was Harlow's experiments (Harlow 1961), carried out under controlled conditions in the laboratory, that compelled the skeptics to take Bowlby's revolutionary ideas seriously.

The problem with Bowlby's conceptual structure was not its limitations but that it explained too much. This problem was, of course, also a strength (and still is) in that it allowed a great many observations in both humans and other animals to be grouped together and integrated within a single powerful idea. But for the psychoanalysts, Bowlby's theory attempted to take over much that was better understood within existing concepts of early appetite, sex, and aggression. For many behavioral scientists studying early development experimentally, evidence from their research did not fit Bowlby's concept of a *unitary* attachment system at work within the mother–infant interaction. Instead, they found several relatively independent systems (e.g., for orientation, for early learning and memory, for thermal regulation, or for early affect expression), each with its own regulatory principles. In addition, Bowlby's concept did not generate research questions but rather seemed to answer questions with a frustrating form of circular reasoning. For example, the strength of an infant's attachment was assessed through the intensity of the response to separation, which itself was explained as the consequence of disruption of the attachment bond.

A resolution of this ambivalence toward the concept of attachment has come in the last decade with major developments in psychoanalysis and in developmental psychobiology. The growth and acceptance of psychoanalytic object relations theory and the advent of parent–infant programs within psychoanalytic institutes have created new forms of treatment and fertile areas for research focused on early attachment. Within the fields of developmental psychobiology and behavioral neuroscience, *attachment* has found a place as a unifying descriptive term for an area of research involving processes at work within close social relationships. Among specific advances in our understanding of the component behavioral processes and neural mechanisms involved in the origin, maintenance, and termination of the attachment between the mammalian infant and its mother, siblings, and father, the idea of a neurobiology of attachment has become more than a figment of the imagination.

I believe that the crucial step that has made a science of attachment possible has been the realization that its psychological constructs could be analyzed at a level of component processes operating at a simpler level of organization. This new way of thinking allowed researchers to generate multiple hypotheses, each of which could be disproved or supported by experiments that gave unambiguous answers. Exploring this level of analysis has been exciting because it does not simply reduce the psychological questions to the most basic elements of biological organization (e.g., cells and molecules), trusting that eventually answers will come from "the bottom up." Rather, this approach focuses on the processes of behavioral organization and regulation that closely underlie psychological constructs, providing a link between psychology and the workings of the brain. New knowledge at this level of analysis seems to deepen our understanding of psychological processes, allowing us to modify our existing higher-level constructs to make them more interesting and useful rather than claiming to eliminate the need for them.

In what follows, I illustrate this approach and how it has helped us to gain a deeper understanding of several features of early attachment that were encompassed by attachment theory but never satisfactorily explained by it. One of John Bowlby's lasting contributions was his placement of attachment in an evolutionary frame and his integration of observations and research with human and animal subjects. He was a great proponent of the value of the study of animal behavior (known as *ethology* at the time), and he saw it as holding out the promise of adding greatly to his insights into human attachment: "With ethological concepts and methods it is possible to undertake a far-reaching program of experimentation into the social responses of the preverbal period of infancy, and to this I attach much importance" (Bowlby 1958, p. 365).

This chapter is organized under the three major aspects of early attachment: 1) the bond, 2) the response to separation, and 3) the long-term effects of the early relationship. Under each of these headings, a series of questions are posed, questions that new research in developmental psychobiology is beginning to answer:

1. Under the concept of a "bond," we asked: How early does the infant know his or her own mother? How does the infant learn to recognize and prefer her? How does the infant develop the ability to orient himself or herself and stay close to his or her mother?
2. Under the concept of response to separation, we asked: What causes the separation response? Why is it so traumatic? What controls the separation cry?
3. Under the concept of long-term effects, we asked: How do qualitatively different early relationships shape later develop-

ment? How are maternal behavior patterns transmitted across generations? How can attachment patterns interact with genetic predispositions to influence long-term outcome?

Finally, this chapter concludes with a summary and an outline of some implications for early human development and for the formation of early mental representations in particular.

The Bond

How Early Does Attachment Begin?

The first strong evidence for fetal learning came from studies on early voice recognition in humans, in which it was found that babies recognize and prefer their own mother's voice, even when tested within hours after birth (DeCasper and Fifer 1980). Fifer continued these studies in our department by using an ingenious device through which newborns could choose between two tape-recorded voices by sucking at different rates on a pacifier rigged to control an audiotape player (reviewed in Fifer and Moon 1995). He found that newborn infants, in the first hours after birth, prefer human voices to silence, female voices to male voices, their native language to another language, and their own mother to another mother reading the same Dr. Seuss story. To obtain more direct evidence for the prenatal origins of these preferences (rather than very rapid postnatal learning), Fifer filtered the high-frequency components from the tapes to make the mother's voice resemble recordings of maternal voice by hydrophones placed within the amniotic space of pregnant women. This altered recording, in which the words were virtually unrecognizable to adults, was preferred to the standard mothers' voice by newborns in the first hours after birth, a preference that tended to wane in the second and third postnatal days. Furthermore, evidence now shows that newborns prefer familiar speech and music sequences to which they have been repeatedly exposed prenatally.

In a striking interspecies similarity, rat pups were shown to discriminate and prefer their own dams' amniotic fluid over that of another dam (Hepper 1987). Newborn pups also required amniotic fluid on a teat in order to find and attach to it for their first nursing attempt (Blass 1990). Robinson and Smotherman (1995) directly tested the hypothesis that pups begin to learn about their mothers' scent in utero and explored the neural substrates for this very early form of plasticity. They used intraoral cannula infusions and perioral stimulation in one trial to show taste aversion learning and classical conditioning in late-term rat fetuses. Taste aversions learned in utero were expressed in the free feeding responses of weanling rats nearly 3 weeks later. They went on to determine that aversive responses to vibrissa stimulation were attenuated or blocked by intraoral milk infusion, a prenatal "comfort" effect they found to be mediated by μ opioid receptors.

These forms of fetal learning involving maternal voice in humans and amniotic fluid in rodents appear to play an adaptive role in preparing the infant for its first extrauterine encounter with its mother. They are thus the earliest origins we have yet found for attachment to the mother. Such powerful demonstrations of learning and reward so early in animal development suggest that we have only begun to explore the human potential for intrauterine effects in the origins of attachment.

How Does the Infant Learn to Recognize and Prefer His or Her Own Mother?

Although specific olfactory and/or auditory predispositions toward the infant's own mother may be acquired prenatally, after birth the newborn enters a new world in which contingent events, so important for more advanced forms of learning, are now occurring with great frequency. Sullivan and colleagues (1986a) showed that associating a novel odor with simulated licking of the pup (stroking with a soft brush), after just a few repetitions, resulted in the pup learning to select, approach, and remain close to that odor. Several different kinds of tactile stimulation, even tail pinch and mild electric shock (which the pups tried to escape from), also induced preferences for the associated odor during the first week of postnatal life. However, such strong and clearly aversive tactile stimulation ceased to induce preferences after the first postnatal week and then began to induce avoidance responses during the second week. These results defined a sensitive period for the formation of positive associations reinforced by intense tactile stimulation. We next found that odors conditioned in this way not only produced olfactory preferences in a choice test; when an inert littermate was scented with the odor, it elicited increased active huddling behavior, probing, and pawing and also increased the time the trained pup spent in contact with the target animal (Sullivan et al. 1986b). Thus, the odor came to arouse the same behaviors normally elicited during interaction with the mother.

This rapid learning process resembles imprinting in birds, and because of the effectiveness of even aversive stimulation at an early age, it reminds us of the clinical observation that strong attachments can occur in children of abusive parents. This learning is limited to an early sensitive period, does not require standard reinforcing events, and accommodates even intense levels of stimulation as reinforcing. Cues learned in this way can be highly specific to an identifying maternal feature; they acquire the capacity to elicit states of increased arousal, and they operate at a distance as incentive cues in a motivational system that ensures close proximity of the infant to the mother (Rosenblatt 1983).

This form of early olfactory learning has become a model system for neurochemical and neuroanatomical studies that have established the existence of a distributed memory system involving the amygdala, hippocampus, and thalamocortical systems as well as the olfactory bulb and cortex (Wilson and Sullivan 1994). Norepinephrine appears to play a dual role in this learning, enhancing olfactory system responsiveness during training and supporting later consolidation of the memory. Dopaminergic, serotoninergic, glutamatergic, and γ-aminobutyric acid (GABA) receptors also have been implicated in modulatory roles. Interestingly, the learning and positive associations to aversive stimuli in the first 10 days require intact μ opioid pathways, whereas associations to more gentle stimulation do not (Sullivan et al. 2000).

Bowlby proposed that early specific proximity-seeking behavior in mammals, including humans, would eventually be explained by the discovery of an early imprinting-like process. It would appear that these results in rat pups identify just such a process.

How Does the Infant Develop the Ability to Orient and Stay Close to the Mother?

In the late prenatal period, rat pups engage in several spontaneous behaviors in utero, including curls, stretches, and trunk and limb turning movements. These acts increased markedly in frequency with progressive removal of intrauterine space constraints as pups were observed first through the uterine wall, then through the thin amniotic sac, and finally in a warm saline bath (Smotherman and Robinson 1986). Recently, Jon Polan and I found that in the first 1–2 hours after birth, pups showed high levels of these same behaviors, regardless of whether they were with their mothers. After the first day's nursing interaction, however, pups' responses became increasingly selective, so that by 2 days postnatal, pups responded in this way only to a lactating dam's ventrum, lowered down over them from above. Their behaviors included the curling and stretching seen prenatally but now also included movement toward the suspended surface, wriggling, audible vocalizations, and, most strikingly, turning upside down toward the surface above them (Polan et al. 2002).

Evidently, these behaviors propel the pup into close contact with the ventrum, maintain it in proximity, and keep it oriented toward the surface. Thus, they appear to be very early orienting and attachment behaviors. In a series of experiments, we found that these are not stereotyped reflex acts, but organized responses that are graded according to the number of maternal modalities present on the surface (e.g., texture, warmth, odor). Furthermore, they are enhanced by periods of prior maternal deprivation, suggesting a motivational component. By age 2 days, we found that pups discriminated their own mother's odor in preference to equally familiar nest odors (Polan and Hofer 1998), and by the first week postnatal, Hepper (1986) showed that pups discriminate and prefer their own mother, father, and siblings to other lactating females, males, or age mates.

These results show that a behavioral attachment system capable of approach and proximity maintenance to the mother, and motivated by brief periods of separation from her, may occur much earlier in development than previously supposed. The remarkable specificity of the approach response of the infant rat to individual family members within the first few postnatal days indicates that specificity of attachment does not require long experience or advanced cognitive and emotional capabilities. Olfaction in the rat and vision in the human provide the necessary basis for approach responses that are specific to a single individual. But this remarkable capability can develop independently of the specificity of its comfort response. Even a 2-week-old pup will show an equal comfort response with any available female. This nonspecificity is limited, however, because 2- to 3-week-old pups clearly avoid the odor of unfamiliar males (but not of familiar males) and show a fear response (immobility) when exposed to them (Takahashi 1992).

Recent work in humans, inspired by these findings in lower animals, has shown that human newborns also are capable of slowly locomoting across the bare surface of the mother's abdomen and locating the breast scented with amniotic fluid in preference to the untreated breast (Varendi et al. 1996). Apparently, human newborns are not as helpless as previously thought and possess specific olfactory approach and orienting behaviors that greatly anticipate the recognized onset of maternal attachment at 6–8 months.

Separation and Loss

How Does Early Separation Exert Its Effects?

Soon after birth, prenatally acquired perceptual biases, stimulus-guided tactile responses, and associative learning create a powerful behavioral control system through which the infant maintains close proximity to his or her mother. However, another important attribute of attachment, by which an emotional tie of the infant to his or her mother has been inferred, is the response to separation. This separation response has been thought to be an integral part of the proximity-maintenance system, one that represents the affective expression of its motivational nature. Thus, the degree or strength of attachment is thought to be responsible for the intensity of the response to separation, and the separation response itself is taken to represent a full expression of the attachment behaviors in the absence of their "goal object" (Bowlby 1969).

Experiments in our laboratory led us to a very different view, in which the processes underlying attachment and the responses to separation are seen as separate and distinct early in life (Hofer 1975a, 1983). The response of infant rats, and primates, to maternal separation has been found to involve a complex pattern of changes in several different behavioral and physiological systems (Hofer 1996b; Kraemer 1992). We found that this pattern was not an integrated psychophysiological response, as had been supposed, but the result of a novel mechanism. During separation, each of the individual systems of the infant rat responded to the absence of one or another of the components of the infant's previous interaction with its mother. Providing one of these components to a separated pup (e.g., maternal warmth) maintained the level of brain biogenic amine function underlying the pup's general activity level (Hofer 1980; Stone et al. 1976) but had no effect on other systems, such as the pup's cardiac rate. Heart rate declined 40% after 18 hours of separation, regardless of whether supplemental heat was provided (Hofer 1971). The heart rate, normally maintained by sympathetic tone, was regulated by maternal provision of milk to neural receptors in the lining of the pup's stomach (Hofer and Weiner 1975). By studying other systems, such as those controlling sleep-wake states (Hofer 1976), activity level (Hofer 1975b), sucking pattern (Brake et al. 1982), vocalization (Hofer and Shair 1980), and blood pressure (Shear et al. 1983), we concluded that in maternal separation, all of the relatively independent regulatory components of the mother–infant interaction were withdrawn at once, yielding a pattern of increases or decreases in levels of function of the infant's systems, depending on whether a particular system had been up- or downregulated by the previous mother–infant interaction. Other investigators who used this approach identified other regulating systems of this sort.

For example, removal of the dam from rat pups was found to produce a rapid (30-minute) decline in the pup's growth hormone (GH) levels, and vigorous tactile stroking of maternally separated pups (mimicking maternal licking) prevented the decrease in GH (reviewed by Kuhn and Schanberg 1991). Brain substrates for this effect were then investigated, and it appears that GH levels are normally maintained by maternal licking, acting through serotonin 2A and 2C receptor modulation of the balance between secretion of hypothalamic GH releasing factor and somatostatin, an inhibitory factor, that together act on the anterior pituitary release of GH (Katz et al. 1996). The withdrawal of maternal licking by separation allows the balance to shift toward somatostatin, resulting in a precipitate decrease in GH.

Several biological similarities are seen between this maternal deprivation effect in rats and the reactive attachment disorder of infancy. Applying this knowledge to prematurely born infants with low birth weights, Field and colleagues (1986) joined the Schanberg group in a landmark study that has since been replicated by others. They used a combination of stroking and limb movement, administered three times a day for 15 minutes each time and continued throughout their 2-week hospitalization. This intervention increased weight gain, head circumference, and behavior development test scores in relation to a randomly chosen control group, with beneficial effects discernible many months later (Field et al. 1986). These infants were able to leave the intensive care unit several days earlier than the control group, which saved thousands of dollars in hospitalization and showed the potential cost-effectiveness of translational research.

What Controls the Separation Cry?

One of the best known responses to maternal separation is the infant's isolation call, a behavior that occurs in a wide variety of species (Lester and Boukydis 1985; Newman 1998). In the rat, this call is in the ultrasonic range (40 kHz) and appears on the first or second postnatal day. Pharmacological studies show that the ultrasonic vocalization response to isolation is attenuated or blocked in a dose-dependent manner by clinically effective anxiolytics that act at benzodiazepine and serotonin receptors. Conversely, ultrasonic vocalization rates are increased by compounds known to be anxiogenic in humans, such as benzodiazepine receptor inverse agonists (β-carboline, FG 1742) and $GABA_A$ receptor ligands such as pentylenetetrazol (Hofer 1996a; Miczek et al. 1991). Within serotonin and opioid systems, receptor subtypes known to have opposing effects on experimental anxiety in adult rats also have opposing effects on infant calling rates. Neuroanatomical studies in infant rats showed that stimulation of the periaqueductal gray area produces ultrasonic vocalization, and chemical lesions of this area prevent calling (Goodwin and Barr 1998). The more distal motor pathway is through the nucleus ambiguus and both laryngeal branches of the vagus nerve. Higher centers known to be involved in cats and primates suggest a neural substrate for isolation calls involving primarily the hypothalamus, amygdala, thalamus, and hippocampus, brain areas known to be involved in adult human and adult animal anxiety and/or defensive responses.

This evidence strongly suggests that separation produces an early affective state in rat pups, which is expressed by the rate of infant calling. How does this calling behavior, and its inferred underlying affective state, develop as a communication system between mother and pup? Infant rat ultrasonic vocalizations are a powerful stimulus for the lactating rat, capable of causing her to interrupt an ongoing nursing bout, initiate searching outside the nest, and direct her search toward the source of the calls (Smotherman et al. 1978). The mother's retrieval response to the pup's vocal signals then results in renewed contact between pup and mother. This contact quiets the pup. The isolation and comfort responses in attachment theory are described as expressions of interruption and reestablishment of a social bond. Such a formulation would predict that because the pup recognizes its mother by her scent (as described earlier), pups made acutely anosmic would fail to show a comfort response. However, anosmic pups show comfort responses that are virtually unaffected by loss of their capacity to recognize their mother in this way (Hofer and Shair 1991). Instead, we and others have found multiple regulators of infant ultrasonic vocalization within the contact between mother and pup: warmth, tactile stimuli, and milk, as well as her scent (Hofer 1996b). Provision of stimulation in these modalities separately (e.g., artificial fur lacking warmth or scent) and then progressively combining them elicits a graded response, with the full comfort response being elicited when all modalities were presented together and maximum calling rates occurring when all were withdrawn at once. In essence, we found parallel regulatory systems involving different sensory modalities. These function in a cumulative or additive way, and the rate of infant calling reflects the sum total of the effective regulatory stimuli present at any given point in time.

After the first postnatal week, a more complex vocal response begins to emerge (Hofer et al. 1998). The pup now begins to regulate its isolation calling response in relation to social cues that were present *before* isolation. If the 2-week-old pup had been with its mother briefly (1–10 minutes) before separation, it called at three to four times the rate typically found after having been in the company of its littermates. If the pup was isolated after having been with a virgin female, or after contact with its mother when she was entirely passive (anesthetized), the pup called at an intermediate rate (Hofer et al. 1999). If, on the other hand, the pup had previously encountered the smell of an unfamiliar adult male (a potential predator) before isolation, it suppressed all vocalization and became immobile when alone (Shair et al. 1997). This silence and stillness could be viewed as a "fear" response, based on prediction of a specific threat, as contrasted with the less well-defined dangers inherent in isolation.

We called the maternal effect *potentiation* and found that the capacity to elicit this response from pups can be acquired by virgin females and even by adult males if the pups have been reared with either adult in addition to their dam prior to testing at age 12 days postnatal (Brunelli et al. 1998). In current research, we are trying to determine exactly what early developmental interactions with the pup these adults must have in order for the pups to later respond to separation from them with a potentiated separation cry.

We hypothesize that this maternal potentiation of the separation cry is a form of affect regulation that may have a human analogy. For example, when a mother returns briefly to the daycare center after dropping off her son to retrieve something she forgot, she is likely to be greeted by an unexpected storm of vocal protest from her toddler as she departs, a much more intense response than when she first dropped him off at the center earlier that morning. A psychological mechanism for this effect is suggested by some interesting learning experiments in rat pups. It was found that 12-day-old rats trained in a runway vocalize at greatly increased rates when their learned expectancy of reward (by maternal contact) was first violated by removal of the dam from the goal box (Amsel et al. 1977). The toddler may expect the mother to take him home when she returns, and the violation of this expectancy produces his vocal outburst.

In summary, in the development of interactions between the infant rat and its mother, a vocal communication system becomes established. The infant separation call rate appears to be controlled by the same neural systems that mediate anxiety in adult animals and humans, apparently a strongly conserved response system. Early in development, the system is regulated simply by the multiple components of the infants' immediate social interaction or by their withdrawal in separation. Later in development, the system comes to be regulated also by traces of the infants' recent past experience with specific social cues that may predict the risk-to-benefit ratio of the calling response attracting predators or eliciting a rapid maternal response.

Long-Term Effects

How Do Early Relationships Shape Later Development?

The actions of maternal regulators of infant biology and behavior are not limited to the mediation of responses to maternal separation discussed in the previous sections. They exert their regulatory effects continuously, throughout the preweaning period and even beyond. A good illustration is the recent discovery of a major role for the mother–infant interaction in the development of the hypothalamic-pituitary-adrenocortical axis (HPA). In mid-infancy, from postnatal days 4 to 14, the rat pups' HPA response to isolation and to mild stressors such as saline injections is less intense than in the newborn or weaning periods, a stage known as the *stress-hyporesponsive period*. Surprisingly, it was recently found that this species-typical developmental stage is not the product of an intrinsic developmental program but the result of hidden regulators at work within the ongoing mother–infant interaction.

First, it was found that 9- to 12-day-old pups' basal cortico-sterone level and the magnitude of the corticotropin and cortico-sterone response to isolation were increased fivefold after 24 hours of maternal separation (Stanton et al. 1988). Next, by using our concept of hidden regulators, Suchecki et al. (1993) attempted to prevent these separation-induced changes by supplying various components of the mother–infant interaction. They found that re-peated stroking of the separated infants for as little as three 1-minute periods prevented the increase in corticotropin response, and providing milk by cheek cannula during separation prevented the separation-induced blunting of the adrenal corticosterone re-sponse to corticotropin. Tracing these regulatory effects back to brain systems, Levine's group found that stroking (representing maternal licking) regulates the intensity of the c-*fos* messenger RNA (mRNA) response in the paraventricular nucleus of the hy-pothalamus and the corticotropin-releasing hormone (CRH) re-ceptor mRNA expression as well in the paraventricular nucleus, the amygdala, and other limbic system sites (van Oers et al. 1998). Intraorally administered milk, however, regulates glucocorticoid receptor mRNA in the CA1 region of the hippocampus and corti-costerone release from the adrenal in response to corticotropin.

Through this anatomical neuromodulator analysis, Levine and colleagues have found that maternal licking and milk delivery during nursing exerted an unexpected and prolonged attenuating effect on the responsiveness of the HPA axis, creating the stress-hyporesponsive period. This maternal regulatory effect, once es-tablished in the first few postnatal days, continues throughout most of the nursing period, finally declining as weaning occurs from day 15 to 21. These regulatory interactions achieve this effect by increasing the inhibitory feedback from hippocampal glucocor-ticoid receptors and by decreasing the hypothalamic stimulation of corticotropin-releasing factor and corticotropin output. These regulatory effects on the pup's brain can be rapidly reversed by maternal separation.

Based on this evolving story, Plotsky and Meaney (1993) ex-plored the possibility that repeated shorter (3-hour) maternal separations during this developmental period might have effects on the HPA that persisted beyond the preweaning period into adulthood. They found elevated basal corticotropin levels, an increased corticotropin response to mild stress, and elevated CRH mRNA expression in the amygdala in adults that had been repeatedly separated as infants. However, in an interesting twist to the story, Plotsky recently found that it was not the effects of the repeated brief separations on the pups but the effects of the separations on maternal behavior after reunion that exerted the long-range shaping effect on HPA development. If the dams were provided with foster pups during the 3-hour separation period, and the pups continued to be separated repeatedly, the long-term effects on the pups were eliminated (Huot et al. 2004).

These findings suggest that qualitative differences in the mother–infant interaction can act to shape development through altered regulation of infant systems. Meaney and colleagues used a maternal behavior observational approach developed previously in our laboratory (Myers et al. 1989) to directly test this implication of the concept of maternal regulators. They found that dams in their colony that were observed naturally to have high levels of licking, grooming, and the high-arched nursing position reared pups that were later found to have lower than normal HPA axis responsivity to restraint stress as adults, whereas the offspring of dams that naturally showed the lowest levels of these interactions resembled the adults with a history of repeated early maternal separations described earlier (Liu et al. 1997). The group was led to this comparison of different mothering patterns by their studies on the classic "handling" effect, in which pups are briefly removed from the home cage and then returned after a few minutes each day for the first 1–2 weeks of postnatal life. This manipulation, they found, reduced HPA reactivity in adult offspring by causing increased glucocorticoid receptor levels and decreased levels of CRH synthesis in the paraventricular nucleus of the adult hypothalamus. When mother–infant interactions of handled litters were observed, the dams showed increases in licking and grooming and in high-arched nursing position in comparison to control litters, measures Meaney and colleagues (Liu et al. 1997) then used in the natural variation studies described earlier.

How Are Maternal Behavior Patterns Transmitted Across Generations?

These laboratory results show that an intervention that alters the mother–infant interaction pattern also changes the adult fear behavior and physiological response characteristics of the offspring. One of the observations that currently occupies researchers in the human clinical attachment area is how mothers in one generation can pass on to their daughters the tendency to child abuse that the mothers had experienced as infants, a pattern shown in primate cross-fostering studies (reviewed in Suomi 1997). The experiment described above provided a chance to determine whether this transgenerational effect occurs in nonprimate species and to explore how it comes about. By allowing the offspring of the handled litters to rear another generation, this time without handling and under normal laboratory conditions, Meaney and colleagues found that the mother–infant interaction shown by these normally reared progeny resembled the interaction their mothers had been induced to have by handling when they were infants (high licking/ grooming and arched-back nursing [LG/ABN]) rather than the one characteristic of their grandmothers before the handling intervention (low LG/ABN) (Francis et al. 1999). Furthermore, the unmanipulated pups in these litters also grew up to show the adult behaviors and hormonal stress patterns recently acquired by their mothers and typical of offspring of high LG/ABN litters.

What could be the mechanism for the transmission of maternal behavior from one generation to the next? A recent article by the same group (Champagne et al. 2001) showed that females that were more responsive to pups had higher levels of oxytocin not only in an area of the brain known to be central in mediating maternal behavior—the medial preoptic area—but also in other related areas. Moreover, giving a drug that blocks oxytocin receptors to the mothers on the third postpartum day completely eliminated the differences between high and low LG/ABN mothers. Thus, we can infer that the oxytocin-based neural precursors for maternal behavior in the infant can be shaped by the infant's interaction with its mother so that later in adulthood, it will show patterns of maternal behavior that reflect this early experience and that may in turn shape the development of maternal behavior in its offspring in the next generation.

These experiments show the intergenerational transmission of mother–infant interaction patterns and the developmental effect of these interaction patterns on adult behavior and physiology. They provide an animal model for the neurobiological analysis of mechanisms underlying environmental effects on the transgenerational patterns of mothering and an experimental verification of one of the central tenets of present-day human attachment research. From an evolutionary perspective, intragenerational effects may have been selected for their ability to preadapt new mothers to prevailing conditions, a biological precursor of the cultural transmission that provides a parallel developmental mechanism in humans.

How Can Attachment Patterns Interact With Genetic Predisposition?

In 1974, two Czech investigators reported the results of a study in which they cross-fostered at birth the offspring of two different strains of rats that they had selectively bred for high and low aggression toward mice (Flandera and Novakova 1974). On cross-fostering pups between mothers of the two different strains, they found that the traits that emerged in the offspring were those typical of their foster mothers rather than of their own genotype. Because the pups never observed adults interacting with mice, the different traits were transmitted in some other way by the mothers during interaction with their foster pups between birth and weaning. Low-aggression strain pups fostered to high-aggression strain dams showed high levels of aggression (65% of them killed mice) both at age 30 days and at age 90 days. Conversely, pups from the high-aggression strain, when cross-fostered to low-aggression strain mothers, showed minimal levels of mouse killing (12.5%) as adolescents (30 days). However, their genotype gradually emerged as the offspring developed increased levels of aggression by age 90 days (50%). This study is a good example of how selective breeding can exert its effect indirectly, through altering the behavior of the mother toward the pups, as well as through more direct effect on the phenotype of the offspring. Unfortunately, these findings were not further explored to determine the behavioral and brain mechanisms for postnatal transmission of the traits.

A more recent example in which postnatal mechanisms were explored involved spontaneously hypertensive rats (SHR) and their Wistar Kyoto (WKY) progenitor control strain. Cross-fostering of the young of the SHR strain at birth to WKY mothers normalized their adult blood pressure, but the low blood pressure of WKY rats was not increased by cross-fostering them at birth to SHR dams (McCarty et al. 1992). The blood pressure of both strains was unaffected by the fostering manipulation itself within strains, and cross-fostering at various ages within the 3 weeks after birth showed that the sensitive period for the normalization of blood pressure was within the first or second postnatal weeks.

We have explored the possible mechanisms for this maternal effect in a series of studies (summarized in Myers et al. 1992). First, we developed methods for the rapid survey of ongoing mother–infant interactions naturally occurring in the maternity cages of a colony, methods later used by Meaney and his group in the HPA axis studies described earlier. In our study, we learned that although members of each of these inbred strains were genetically identical, interlitter variability was significant both in adult blood pressure and in maternal behavior within each strain, as well as between the two strains. Three maternal behaviors accounted for most of the variability in adult blood pressure, both between litters and between strains. Pups of mothers that showed more of these behaviors had higher blood pressure as adults.

By looking carefully at the components of maternal behavior that were most highly correlated with adult blood pressure of the offspring (high-arched nursing position, contact time, and licking), we then made an educated guess that led us to the next chapter in the story. First, we examined the milk letdown that occurred during the high-arched maternal nursing position. We found a sudden transient rise in blood pressure of 50% during natural and oxytocin-induced milk ejection, a greater increase than during any other pup activity (Shair et al. 1986). This surge in blood pressure was caused by a major increase in neural activity in the adrenergic vasoconstrictor system that controls blood vessel tone throughout the body. Shair and Hofer (1993) then found that this surge was triggered by contact of the milk with sensory nerve endings on the tongue and in the throat. Myers et al. (1992) went on to show that the rate of weight gain during a critical period of nursing is a powerful correlate of adult blood pressure and that experimentally increasing the level of milk let-down events, during this 4-day period, by a temporary reduction in litter size significantly increased adult blood pressure of the offspring. The importance of these studies was further increased when Myers and his colleagues found that human infants also show major increases in blood pressure in response to maternal milk letdown (Cohen et al. 1992).

In these studies, the differing adult phenotypic traits of genetically selected lines of laboratory animals have been powerfully shaped (or even determined in the case of mouse killing behavior) by the particular maternal environment in which they were reared as pups. We are beginning to work out the behavioral mechanisms by which specific components of the mother–infant interaction exert these shaping effects on the expression of the genotype through development.

Summary and Implications for Human Development

The research approaches described in this chapter have begun to answer the three questions posed in the beginning of this chapter: 1) How does the infant first acquire the propensity to maintain close contact with his or her caregiver? 2) Why does interruption of this contact produce such extensive biological and behavioral responses in the offspring? and 3) How do seemingly minor variations in the ongoing patterns of the mother–infant interaction become translated into long-term differences between individuals in adulthood, even extending to the next generation? Until recently, we have attempted to answer these questions primarily in terms of inferred motivational and emotional states maturing in the infant and child. Attachment has been viewed as a unified system, separate from other motivational systems. The complex response to separation has been seen as an emotional response expressing high levels of this motivational state, and the long-term effects that follow variations in the quality of the early mother–infant relationship were believed to reflect persistent differences induced in emotion regulation within the maturing attachment system.

The new work outlined in this chapter indicates a level of developmental process that underlies these inferred emotional responses and that provides a different kind of explanation for the observed responses of the infant. These processes act at a sensorimotor and physiological level that translates readily to the level of neural events and opens up the potential for us to understand how these emotional states become organized in the developing brain of the infant.

From Regulation to Representation

The early learning and widespread regulatory interactions described above are not involved solely in biological and behavioral development but are also the first experiences out of which mental representations and their associated emotions arise in human development. So far, as we understand the process, experiences consisting of the infant's individual acts, parental responses, sensory impressions, and associated affects are set in memory during and after early parent–infant interactions. These individual units of experience are integrated into something like a network of attributes in memory, invested with associated affect, and result in the formation of an internal working model of the relationship. In this way, the learning and regulatory interactions we have described in infancy become ingredients for the mental representations and related affective qualities that form the inner experience of older children and adults (D.N. Stern 1985). Once formed, it seems likely that these organized mental structures come to act as superordinate regulators of behavioral and biological systems underlying motivation and affect, gradually supplanting the sensorimotor, thermal, and nutrient regulatory systems found in younger infants. These developmental processes would link biological systems with internal object representations in humans and would account for the remarkable upheavals of biological as well as psychological systems that occur in adults in response to cues signaling impending separation or in response to losses established simply on hearing of a death, for example, by telephone (Hofer 1984).

Mother–infant relationships that differ in quality and that necessarily involve different levels and patterns of regulation in a variety of systems will be reflected in the nature of the mental representations present in different children as they grow up. The emotions aroused during early crying responses to separation, during the profound state changes associated with the prolonged loss of all maternal regulators, and during the reunion of a separated infant with his or her mother are clearly intense. These emotional states have commanded our attention; they are what everyone intuitively recognizes about attachment and separation and what we feel about the people we are close to. These inner experiences occur at a different level of psychobiological organization than the changes in autonomic, endocrine, and neurophysiological systems we have been able to study in rats and monkeys, as well as in younger human infants.

Later Regulatory Interactions

The discovery of early maternal regulatory interactions and the effects of their withdrawal allow us to understand not only the responses to separation in young organisms of limited cognitive-emotional capacity but also the familiar experienced emotions and memories that can be verbally described to us by older children and adults. It is not that rat pups respond only to loss of maternal regulators, whereas human infants respond to loss with complex emotions of love, sadness, anger, and grief. Human infants, as they mature, can respond at the symbolic level *as well as* at the level of the behavioral and physiological processes of the regulatory interactions. The two levels appear to be organized as parallel and complementary response systems. Even *adult* humans continue to respond in important ways at the sensorimotor–physiological level in their social interactions, separations, and losses, continuing a process begun in infancy. A good example of this sensorimotor–physiological response is the mutual regulation of menstrual synchrony among close female friends, an effect that takes place out of conscious awareness and has been found to be mediated at least in part by a pheromonal cue (K. Stern and McClintock 1998). Other examples may well include the role of social interactions in entraining circadian physiological rhythms and the remarkable effects of social support on the course of medical illness (Hofer 1984). In this way, adult love, grief, and bereavement may well contain elements of the simpler regulatory processes that we can clearly see in the attachment responses of infant animals to separation from their social companions.

The concept of regulation as inherent in the mother–infant interaction in humans now has widespread use. It is generally used in two ways: 1) to refer to the graded effects of different patterns of interaction on the emotional responses of the infant, the so-called regulation of affect (Schore 1994), and 2) to refer to how the behaviors initiated by the infant or mother and their responses to each other act to regulate the interaction itself, its tempo or rhythm (hence, its quality), or the distance (both psychological and physical) between the members of the dyad. The word *regulation* is probably overused currently and inappropriately applied to any influence of one member of the dyad on the other.

Implications for Intervention

First, we should analyze the interactive mechanisms of early developmental regulation in greater detail at the behavioral and physiological levels in animal and human infants to identify the component processes underlying the effects. This level of understanding should lead to novel and unexpected intervention strategies such as those described earlier in this chapter by Field and colleagues (1986).

Second, we should continue to expand the focus of intervention efforts on a broader range of the infant's cognitive and emotional processes, with more emphasis on interactions with the mother that fall outside the traditional categories of attachment behavior.

Third, we need to look for ways to intervene earlier in development and experiment with interactions that involve multiple sensory systems of the infant and use simple biological interactions involving touch, warmth, smell, oral stimulation, and the senses of position and motion of limbs and body in space.

Fourth, we should increase our attention on the maternal side of the interaction rather than on finding new artificial early-stimulation toys for the infant. The mother's environment *outside* of her relationship with the infant should be explored as a means of altering her interaction *with* her infant. In the mother–infant interaction, we must think of new ways to alter how the infant affects the mother rather than concentrating on how the mother affects her infant.

Finally, above all, we should question our preconceptions, try new things out, and think broadly of the mother and the infant developing together rather than limiting our thinking to the boundaries of our current model of attachment.

References

Amsel A, Radek CC, Graham M, et al: Ultrasound emission in infant rats as an indicant of arousal during appetitive learning and extinction. Science 197:786–788, 1977

Blass EM: Suckling: determinants, changes, mechanisms, and lasting impressions. Dev Psychol 26:520–533, 1990

Bowlby J: The nature of the child's tie to his mother. Int J Psychoanal 39:350–373, 1958

Bowlby J: Attachment and Loss, Vol 1: Attachment. New York, Basic Books, 1969

Brake SC, Sager DJ, Sullivan R, et al: The role of intraoral and gastrointestinal cues in the control of sucking and milk consumption in rat pups. Dev Psychobiol 15:529–541, 1982

Brunelli SA, Masmela JR, Shair HN, et al: Effects of biparental rearing on ultrasonic vocalization (USV) responses of rat pups (Rattus norvegicus). J Comp Psychol 112:331–343, 1998

Champagne F, Diorio J, Sharma S, et al: Naturally occurring variations in maternal behavior in the rat are associated with differences in estrogen-inducible central oxytocin receptors. Proc Natl Acad Sci U S A 98:12736–12741, 2001

Cohen M, Witherspoon M, Brown DR, et al: Blood pressure increases in response to feeding in the term neonate. Dev Psychobiol 25:291–298, 1992

DeCasper AJ, Fifer WP: Of human bonding: newborns prefer their mothers' voices. Science 208:1174–1176, 1980

Field TM, Schanberg SM, Scafidid F, et al: Tactile/kinesthetic stimulation effects on preterm neonates. Pediatrics 77:654–658, 1986

Fifer WP, Moon CM: The effects of fetal experience with sound, in Fetal Development—A Psychobiological Perspective. Edited by Lecanuet J-P, Fifer WP, Krasnegor NA, et al. Hillsdale, NJ, Lawrence Erlbaum, 1995, pp 351–368

Flandera V, Novakova V: Effect of mother on the development of aggressive behavior in rats. Dev Psychobiol 8:49–54, 1974

Francis D, Diorio J, Liu D, et al: Nongenomic transmission across generations of maternal behavior and stress responses in the rat. Science 186:1155–1158, 1999

Goodwin GA, Barr GA: Behavioral and heart rate effects of infusing of kainic acid into the dorsal midbrain during early development in the rat. Brain Res Dev Brain Res 107:11–20, 1998

Harlow HF: The development of affectional patterns in infant monkeys, in Determinants of Infant Behaviour, Vol 1. Edited by Foss BM. London, Methuen, 1961, pp 75–88

Heim C, Nemeroff CB: The role of childhood trauma in the neurobiology of mood and anxiety disorders: preclinical and clinical studies. Biol Psychiatry 49:1023–1039, 2001

Hepper PG: Kin recognition: functions and mechanisms, a review. Biol Rev Camb Philos Soc 61:63–93, 1986

Hepper PG: The amniotic fluid: an important priming role in kin recognition. Anim Behav 35:1343–1346, 1987

Hofer MA: Cardiac rate regulated by nutritional factor in young rats. Science 172:1039–1041, 1971

Hofer MA: Infant separation responses and the maternal role. Biol Psychiatry 10:149–153, 1975a

Hofer MA: Studies on how early maternal separation produces behavioral change in young rats. Psychosom Med 37:245–264, 1975b

Hofer MA: The organization of sleep and wakefulness after maternal separation in young rats. Dev Psychobiol 9:189–205, 1976

Hofer MA: The effects of reserpine and amphetamine on the development of hyperactivity in maternally deprived rat pups. Psychosom Med 42:513–520, 1980

Hofer MA: On the relationship between attachment and separation processes in infancy, in Emotions in Early Development. Edited by Plutchik R, Kellerman H. New York, Academic Press, 1983, pp 199–216

Hofer MA: Relationships as regulators: a psychobiological perspective on bereavement. Psychosom Med 46:183–197, 1984

Hofer MA: Multiple regulators of ultrasonic vocalization in the infant rat. Psychoneuroendocrinology 21:203–217, 1996a

Hofer MA: On the nature and consequences of early loss. Psychosom Med 58:570–581, 1996b

Hofer MA, Shair HN: Sensory processes in the control of isolation-induced ultrasonic vocalization by 2-week-old rats. J Comp Physiol Psychol 94:271–299, 1980

Hofer MA, Shair HN: Trigeminal and olfactory pathways mediating isolation distress and companion comfort responses in rat pups. Behav Neurosci 105:699–706, 1991

Hofer MA, Weiner H: Physiological mechanisms for cardiac control by nutritional intake after early maternal separation in the young rat. Psychosom Med 37:8–24, 1975

Hofer MA, Masmela JR, Brunelli SA, et al: The ontogeny of maternal potentiation of the infant rats' isolation call. Dev Psychobiol 33:189–201, 1998

Hofer MA, Masmela JR, Brunelli SA, et al: Behavioral mechanisms for active maternal potentiation of isolation calling in rat pups. Behav Neurosci 113:51–61, 1999

Huot RL, Gonzalez ME, Ladd CO, et al: Foster litters prevent hypothalamic-pituitary-adrenal axis sensitization mediated by neonatal maternal separation. Psychoneuroendocrinology 29:279–289, 2004

Katz LM, Nathan L, Kuhn CM, et al: Inhibition of GH in maternal separation may be mediated through altered serotonergic activity at $5HT_{2A}$ and $5HT_{2C}$ receptors. Psychoneuroendocrinology 21:219–235, 1996

Kraemer GW: A psychobiological theory of attachment. Behav Brain Sci 15:493–511, 1992

Kuhn CM, Schanberg SM: Stimulation in infancy and brain development, in Psychopathology and the Brain. Edited by Carroll BJ, Barrett JE. New York, Raven, 1991

Lester BM, Boukydis CF (eds): Infant Crying: Theoretical and Research Perspectives. New York, Plenum, 1985

Liu D, Diorio J, Tannenbaum B, et al: Maternal care, hippocampal glucocorticoid receptors, and hypothalamic-pituitary-adrenal responses to stress. Science 277:1659–1661, 1997

Margolis G, Gordis EB: The effects of family and community violence on children. Annu Rev Psychol 51:445–479, 2002

McCarty R, Cierpial MA, Murphy CA, et al: Maternal involvement in the development of cardiovascular phenotype. Experientia 48:315–322, 1992

Miczek KA, Tornatsky W, Vivian J: Ethology and neuropharmacology: rodent ultrasounds, in Advances in Pharmacologic Sciences. Basel, Switzerland, Birkhauser, 1991, pp 409–429

Myers MM, Brunelli SA, Squire JM, et al: Maternal behavior of SHR rats in its relationship to offspring blood pressure. Dev Psychobiol 22:29–53, 1989

Myers MM, Shair HN, Hofer MA: Feeding in infancy: short and long-term effects on cardiovascular function. Experientia 48:322–333, 1992

Newman JD (ed): The Physiological Control of Mammalian Vocalization. New York, Plenum, 1998

Plotsky PM, Meaney MJ: Early postnatal experience alters hypothalamic corticotropin-releasing factor (CRF) mRNA: median eminence CRF content and stress-induced release in rats. Brain Res Mol Brain Res 18:195–200, 1993

Polan HJ, Hofer MA: Olfactory preference for mother over home nest shavings by newborn rats. Dev Psychobiol 33:5–20, 1998

Polan HJ, Milano D, Eljuga L, et al: Development of rats: maternally directed orienting behaviors from birth to day 2. Dev Psychobiol 40:81–103, 2002

Robinson SR, Smotherman WP: Habituation and classical conditioning in the rat fetus: opioid involvements, in Fetal Development—A Psychobiological Perspective. Edited by Lecanuet J-P, Fifer WP, Krasnegor NA, et al. Hillsdale, NJ, Lawrence Erlbaum, 1995, pp 295–314

Rosenblatt JS: Olfaction mediates developmental transition in the altricial newborn of selected species of mammals. Dev Psychobiol 16:347–375, 1983

Schore AN: Affect Regulation and the Origin of the Self. Hillsdale, NJ, Lawrence Erlbaum, 1994

Shair HN, Hofer MA: Afferent control of pressor responses to feeding in young rats. Physiol Behav 53:565–576, 1993

Shair HN, Brake SC, Hofer MA, et al: Blood pressure responses to milk ejection in the young rat. Physiol Behav 37:171–176, 1986

Shair HN, Masmela JR, Brunelli SA, et al: Potentiation and inhibition of ultrasonic vocalization of rat pups: regulation by social cues. Dev Psychobiol 30:95–200, 1997

Shear MK, Brunelli SA, Hofer MA: The effects of maternal deprivation and of refeeding on the blood pressure of infant rats. Psychosom Med 45:3–9, 1983

Smotherman WP, Robinson SR: Environmental determinants of behaviour in the rat fetus. Anim Behav 34:1859–1873, 1986

Smotherman WP, Bell RW, Hershberger WA, et al: Orientation to rat pup cues: effects of maternal experiential history. Anim Behav 26:265–273, 1978

Stanton MD, Gutierrez YR, Levine S: Maternal deprivation potentiates pituitary-adrenal stress responses in infant rats. Behav Neurosci 102:692–700, 1988

Stern DN: The Interpersonal World of the Infant: A View From Psychoanalysis and Developmental Psychology. New York, Basic Books, 1985

Stern K, McClintock MK: Regulation of ovulation by human pheromones. Nature 392:177–179, 1998

Stone E, Bonnet K, Hofer MA: Survival and development of maternally deprived rats: role of body temperature. Psychosom Med 33:242–249, 1976

Suchecki D, Rosenfeld P, Levine S: Maternal regulation of the hypothalamic-pituitary-adrenal axis in the infant rat: the roles of feeding and stroking. Brain Res Dev Brain Res 75:185–192, 1993

Sullivan RM, Brake SC, Hofer MA, et al: Huddling and independent feeding of neonatal rats can be facilitated by a conditioned change in behavioral state. Dev Psychobiol 19:625–635, 1986a

Sullivan RM, Hofer MA, Brake SC: Olfactory-guided orientation in neonatal rats is enhanced by a conditioned change in behavioral state. Dev Psychobiol 19:615–623, 1986b

Sullivan RM, Landers M, Yeager B, et al: Good memories of bad events in infancy. Nature 407:38–39, 2000

Suomi SJ: Early determinants of behaviour: evidence from primate studies. Br Med Bull 53:170–184, 1997

Takahashi LK: Developmental expression of defensive responses during exposure to nonspecific adults in preweanling rats (Rattus norvegicus). J Comp Psychol 106:69–77, 1992

van Oers HJJ, de Kloet ER, Whelan T, et al: Maternal deprivation effect on the infant's neural stress markers is reversed by tactile stimulation and feeding but not by suppressing corticosterone. J Neurosci 18:10171–10179, 1998

Varendi H, Porter RH, Winberg J: Attractiveness of amniotic fluid odor: evidence of prenatal olfactory learning? Acta Paediatr 85:1223–1227, 1996

Wilson DA, Sullivan RM: Neurobiology of associative learning in the neonate: early olfactory learning. Behav Neural Biol 61:1–18, 1994

Chapter 2

Developmental Neurobiology of Face Processing

Lisa S. Scott, B.S.
Charles A. Nelson, Ph.D.

Several lines of research suggest that face processing is a "special" perceptual ability that is subserved by a distinct neural system (Haxby et al. 2001; Kanwisher et al. 1997). Furthermore, face perception has been cited as the most developed visual-perceptual skill in humans (Haxby et al. 2000). Indeed, several researchers have claimed that adult face processing can be characterized as a uniquely expert system in humans (Gauthier and Tarr 1997). The extant literature on the basic organization and neural underpinnings of adult face processing is riddled with controversy and may be better informed by an understanding of the processes involved in the development of this system. The fundamental question of how a perceptual system *becomes* functionally and structurally specialized has great potential to inform us about the basic characteristics of that perceptual system and how it came into being.

Many investigators who study face processing in adults view faces as a "special" class of perceptual stimuli. This view is gener-

Support for the writing of this chapter was provided to Dr. Nelson by the National Institutes of Health (NS329976) and by the John D. and Catherine T. MacArthur Foundation through their support of a research network on *Early Experience and Brain Development* and to Lisa Scott from a training grant provided by the National Institute of Child Health and Human Development to the Center for Cognitive Sciences at the University of Minnesota (5T32 HD07151).

ally taken to mean that the mechanisms underlying face processing differ from those underlying the processing of nonface objects. Indeed, behavioral, neuropsychological, and neuroimaging data from patient populations support the existence of a "face module." The special nature of face processing compared with other types of visual processing, such as object processing, originates from reports of patients who are unable to recognize familiar faces but who maintain the ability to recognize and identify objects (Damasio et al. 1982; De Renzi 1986) and from single-cell recordings from nonhuman primates that suggest that cells within the inferior temporal cortex fire preferentially to faces (Gross et al. 1969, 1972; Perrett et al. 1982, 1987).

Although it is beyond the scope of this chapter to provide a comprehensive review of the adult face-processing literature, we refer the interested reader to several relevant articles (Gauthier et al. 1998, 1999a, 2000; Haxby et al. 2000, 2001; Kanwisher et al. 1997). In this chapter, we focus on studies that have investigated the neural and behavioral development of the face-processing system, including studies that have investigated face perception in children with disorders such as autism. Finally, we conclude with a discussion of current models of the development of face processing and how these models inform the study of face processing as a whole.

Neural Correlates of Face Processing in Developmental Populations

Although our understanding of developmental science has greatly benefited from studies investigating the behavioral correlates of development, relatively few studies have investigated the neural systems that underlie changes in behavior across time. The merging of the fields of neuroscience and psychology has recently begun to provide researchers with the ability to examine brain–behavior relations from multiple levels of analysis (for elaboration, see Nelson and Bloom 1997; Nelson et al. 2002). Particularly noteworthy have been advances in noninvasive functional imaging of the developing brain. Functional magnetic resonance imaging (fMRI) and event-related potentials (ERPs) are the most commonly used techniques with normative developmental populations. fMRI provides an index of changes in blood oxygenation levels in the brain, and ERPs provide an index of the electric potential directly generated by neuronal activity. fMRI provides excellent spatial resolution of brain metabolism in response to specific stimuli or cognitive tasks. ERPs, on the other hand, have better temporal resolution and are able to record the response of electrical activity (on the order of milliseconds) to different stimuli from the scalp. (For an extensive review of these techniques in the context of development, see M. de Haan and Thomas 2002; DeBoer et al., in press.)

When studying face processing, one needs to take into account several factors that may influence the processing of certain kinds of faces and how this processing is different from other perceptual processing. For example, we should examine the distinction between face and object processing; the role of familiarity; how different species, genders, races, and ages are processed; the difference between configural and featural face processing; and how emotional expressions are processed. The following review of the developmental literature is limited to research that investigated the neural correlates of these different aspects of face processing with both fMRI and ERP, as well as studies of patient populations and children with developmental disorders.

Faces Versus Objects

A fundamental finding in the study of visual processes is the distinction between the visual pathway that analyzes objects and faces (the ventral "what" pathway) and the visual pathway that analyzes spatial information (the dorsal "where" pathway). Although few investigations have examined the development of these pathways, children (ages 10–12 years) have been found to have a more diffuse and distributed area of activation in both the "what" and the "where" pathways compared with adults (Passarotti et al. 2003). More specifically, children, similar to adults, showed more right compared with left fusiform activation in response to faces, but activation in both hemispheres was more distributed across the temporal cortex in children compared with adults (Figure 2–1).

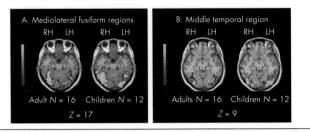

Figure 2–1. Face-matching task.

A: Significant clusters of functional activation in mediolateral fusiform regions for the face-matching task in 16 adults *(left side)* and 12 children *(right side)*. **B:** Significant clusters of functional activation in the middle temporal gyrus in 16 adults *(left side)* and 12 children *(right side)*. Note that according to radiological convention, the left side of the brain represents the right hemisphere, and the right side of the brain represents the left hemisphere. *Source.* Adapted from Passarotti AM, Paul BM, Bussiere JR, et al.: "The Development of Face and Location Processing: An fMRI Study." *Developmental Science* 6:100–117, 2003. Used with permission from Blackwell Publishing.

As with adults, both infants and children show apparent neural dissociations between face and object processing (e.g., Carver et al. 2003; M. de Haan and Nelson 1997, 1999). For example, electrophysiological evidence suggests that certain ERP components differentiate faces and objects. ERPs can be defined as transient changes in the brain's electrical activity that occur in response to a discrete (time-locked) stimulus or an event such as a presentation of a face (M. de Haan and Nelson 1997). ERP components represent negative (denoted by N) and positive (denoted by P) deflections in voltage over time. These components can be either described by the latency of the negative or positive deflection (e.g., N170 is a negative component occurring 170 milliseconds after stimulus onset) or denoted by the number of the positive or negative peak (e.g., a P3 refers to the third positive peak). These deflections are thought to represent different aspects of cognitive and perceptual processing. Several studies with adults have found a negatively peaked component, called the N170, which appears to be highly specific to face processing (for example, Carmel and Bentin 2002). In infants, the P400 component discriminates faces and objects, as evidenced by an earlier latency to peak response to faces in 6-month-olds (M. de Haan and Nelson 1999). This difference is most prominent over posterior and temporal electrode locations, suggesting, similar to findings with adults, a temporal advantage for processing faces. The negative component (Nc), a component associated with attention and recognition memory, is more specific to familiar face stimuli (confined to the midline and right anterior temporal regions) than to familiar object stimuli (distributed across all temporal regions; M. de Haan and Nelson 1999). Furthermore, the Nc is greater in response to familiar objects (e.g., a favorite toy from home), compared with unfamiliar or novel objects. These results suggest differential electrophysiological signatures for objects and faces in 6-month-old infants, which may be related to different levels of experience with specific kinds of object categories (faces vs. objects).

Familiar Versus Unfamiliar Faces

Behavioral studies that used looking time and habituation techniques with newborns reported that infants discriminate between familiar and unfamiliar faces (Pascalis and de Schonen 1994; Pascalis et al. 1995). However, the direction of infants' preference depends on the task used. For example, in a simple visual preference task, infants prefer to look at familiar faces (Pascalis and de Schonen 1994), whereas in studies in which the habituation procedure is used, infants tend to prefer to look at the novel face (Pascalis et al. 1995). Further evidence from electrophysiological investigations indicates that by age 6 months, infants show differential brain activity to familiar (mother's face) and unfamiliar faces (M. de Haan and Nelson 1997, 1999). The Nc has been found to be larger in response to the mother's face than to a stranger's face. This differential activation is influenced by how similar the unfamiliar faces were to the mother's face. This finding, as well as the finding stated earlier with object processing, contrasts with previous research showing a greater Nc to unfamiliar stimuli compared with briefly, or newly, familiarized stimuli (Nelson and Collins 1991). A later positive slow-wave component, maximal over frontal scalp locations and often associated with memory processes (Nelson 1994; Nelson and Monk 2001), was found to discriminate the mother's face from a stranger's face as indexed by a greater response to the stranger's face (M. de Haan and Nelson 1999).

Further research suggests that there may be developmental

changes in the relative importance of viewing different kinds of faces (such as the mother's face vs. strangers' faces). Indeed, children (ages 18–54 months) who were presented with both highly familiar and unfamiliar faces and toys while ERPs were recorded showed changes in only the brain response to faces, and not toys, as a function of age (Carver et al. 2003). More specifically, all age groups showed larger Nc and P400 components to unfamiliar compared with familiar objects, but only children between ages 18 and 24 months showed a greater ERP response to the mother's face than to a stranger's face. Children between ages 45 and 54 months showed a larger response to the stranger's face, and children between ages 24 and 45 months did not show a differential response to either stimulus at the Nc. These findings suggest that the neural correlates of face processing may change across development and may be related to the emotional salience or significance of the face.

"Other-Race" and "Other-Species" Effects

Although not yet studied in infants or very young children, the "other-race" effect, a commonly reported experience in which adults describe more difficulty differentiating between faces from races other than their own (Chance et al. 1982; O'Toole et al. 1994), speaks to the role of experience in the development of face processing. Beginning in the late 1960s and continuing through the 1970s, this phenomenon was attributed to greater exposure to faces of your own race than to others (Brigham and Barkowitz 1978; Brigham and Malpass 1985; Malpass and Kravitz 1969). Fallshore and Scholler (1995) showed that recognition of faces of other races is less affected by inversion than recognition of faces of the same race. Imaging studies of the other-race effect show better recognition memory for same-race faces compared with other-race faces that is paralleled by greater activation of the fusiform area in response to same-race faces compared with faces of another race (Golby et al. 2001). Furthermore, the behavioral memory differences between same- and other-race faces correlates with activation in the fusiform and hippocampal areas. The differences in activation found in the fusiform area have been attributed to different levels of expertise or experience with faces of other races.

As stated earlier in this section, no studies have examined this phenomenon in very young children or infants; however, in contrast to Caucasian adults and older children, Caucasian children as young as 6 years do not show a recognition memory advantage for Caucasian compared with Asian faces (Chance et al. 1982).

The other-race effect also has been modeled with computational face recognition algorithms (Furl et al. 2002). Furl and colleagues tested several face recognition algorithms to determine which was most consistent with behavioral results suggesting better recognition accuracy within races compared with across races. Results were consistent with the "developmental contact" hypothesis. Only experience-based models showed the other-race effect, and this effect was seen only when experience warped the perceptual space to enhance encoding distinctions of same-race faces compared with other-race faces (Furl et al. 2002).

Similar to the "other-race" effect, there have been reports of an "other-species" effect. For example, humans and nonhuman primates are better at recognizing faces of their own species (Pascalis and Bachevalier 1998). More specifically, monkeys tend to look longer at novel monkey faces but not novel human faces, and adult humans look longer at novel human faces but not novel monkey faces. This finding suggests a "species-specific" effect in face recognition. Interestingly, the monkeys in this experiment had more experience with human faces than the humans had with monkey faces. Therefore, Pascalis and Bachevalier asserted that if visual experience were solely responsible for the development and specification of this system, then the nonhuman primates in this study should have shown a novelty preference for both human and monkey faces. A somewhat similar dissociation also has been found in the recognition of inverted faces (Pascalis and Bachevalier 1998). Human adults show an inversion effect for human and monkey faces but not for sheep faces, suggesting that primate faces are being processed in a similar manner compared with sheep faces. Furthermore, children (ages 5–8 years), who have less experience with faces than adults do, show a similar pattern of results (Pascalis et al. 2001). In a forced-choice task, older children are better than younger children at recognizing both upright and inverted faces regardless of species. Recognition was better for human faces than for monkey faces and better for human and monkey faces compared to sheep faces at all ages tested. In addition, similar to adult findings, only human and monkey faces induced an inversion effect. Pascalis and colleagues suggested that the human face-processing system may be tuned to the characteristics of primate (human and monkey) faces by age 5 years.

Recently, the visual paired comparison procedure has been used in adults and in infants ages 6–9 months to determine their sensitivity to human versus monkey faces (Pascalis et al. 2002). This study was designed to test directly a model put forth by Nelson (2001, 2003) that hypothesizes a narrowing of perceptual space in face processing and is described later in this chapter, in the section "Developmental Theories of Face Processing." Pascalis et al. (2002) hypothesized that younger infants would have a more broadly tuned face-processing system and should be better than adults and older infants at discriminating between individual faces within and across different species. Results confirmed this hypothesis, indicating that adults and 9-month-old infants looked longer at novel human faces but looked equally long at novel and familiar monkey faces. In contrast, 6-month-old infants showed novelty preferences in both the human and the monkey conditions.

The findings of the study described in the previous paragraph are supported by the results of an electrophysiological study in which ERPs were recorded from adults and 6-month-old infants while they viewed both upright and inverted monkey and human faces (de Haan et al. 2002b). The purpose of this study was to determine whether adults and infants show the same cortical specificity during face processing. In adults, all stimuli evoked an N170 over temporal and occipital leads. This N170 was larger in amplitude and longer in latency for upright monkey faces compared with upright human faces. Furthermore, inversion effects were apparent in the human but not the monkey conditions (increased amplitude and latency to inverted faces). Results indicated that no component of the infant ERP showed the same specificity as the adult N170 (Figure 2–2). Six-month-old infants showed sensitivity to both inversion and species conditions, but it was distributed across two components. The early Nc (260–336 ms) was greater to human than to monkey faces, and a later positive component (P400) was greater for upright compared with inverted faces. These findings suggest that adultlike patterns of face processing are not mature by age 6 months and may reflect a gradual specialization of cortical face-processing systems.

In a follow-up investigation of this study, 3- and 12-month-old infants were shown upright and inverted monkey and human faces while ERPs were recorded to further elucidate the developmental characteristics of the infant face components (Halit et al. 2003). Results indicated that similar to adults, 12-month-old infants had an Nc (N290) that was larger in amplitude and longer in latency for human than for monkey faces. This component also showed an inversion effect, with a larger amplitude response to inverted compared with upright faces (for humans only). The P400 component also differentiated these conditions, as evidenced by a longer latency response to monkey compared with human faces and a longer latency to inverted compared with upright faces. In contrast, similar to the 6-month data reported earlier in this section, 3-month-old infants did not show the same specificity for human faces that 12-month-olds and adults showed. The results of the previously described studies suggested that the adult N170 may be an emergent product of two developmental components (a negative N290 and a P400) and that the specificity of these components may develop some time between age 6 and 12 months.

Results of the study described in the previous paragraph are somewhat consistent with a study ongoing in our laboratory that uses ERPs with adults and 9-month-old infants to examine discrimination of monkey and human faces in both frontal and profile (as opposed to inverted) orientations (Scott and Nelson 2003). This study was designed to investigate further the neural mechanisms underlying the development of face processing. Adult and 9-month-old participants were familiarized to images of monkey or human faces in the frontal orientation posing neutral expressions (Figure 2–3). After familiarization, participants were tested with novel and familiar monkey or human faces, each in a frontal and profile orientation. Preliminary behavioral analyses

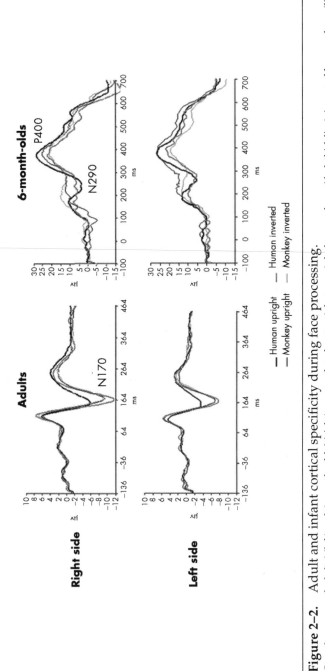

Figure 2–2. Adult and infant cortical specificity during face processing.

Grand average of adults' (*left*) and 6-month-olds' (*right*) event-related potentials to upright human faces (*dark thick line*), inverted human faces (*light thick line*), upright monkey faces (*dark thin line*), and inverted monkey faces (*light thin line*) at the right posterior temporal (T6) and left posterior temporal (T5) electrodes.

Source. Adapted from de Haan M, Pascalis O, Johnson MH: "Specialization of Neural Mechanisms Underlying Face Recognition in Human Infants." *Journal of Cognitive Neuroscience* 12:199–209, 2002b. Copyright 2002 by the Massachusetts Institute of Technology. Used with permission.

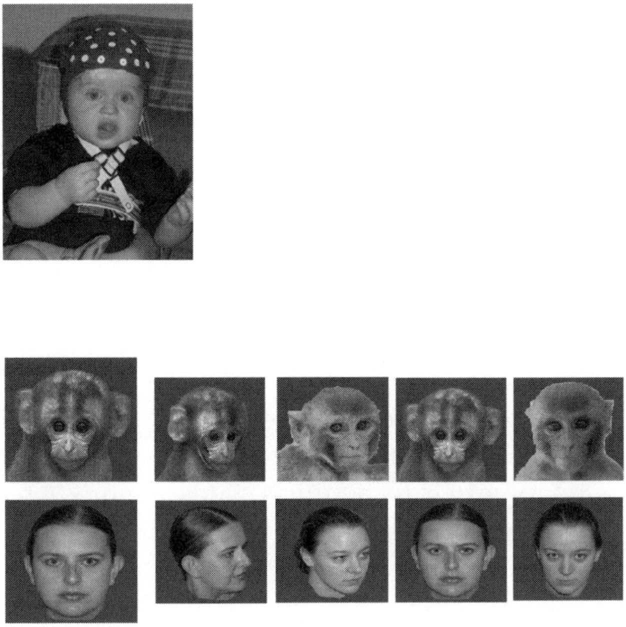

Figure 2–3. Face-processing task.

A: Picture of a 9-month-old infant with a 32-channel electrode cap on his head. **B:** Stimuli used in this task. Infants were first habituated to either one human or one monkey face. Then infants passively viewed serial presentations of the familiar and an unfamiliar face in both frontal and profile orientations.

from adults indicated that participants performed significantly better in the human compared with the monkey discrimination task. Furthermore, preliminary adult ERP analyses indicated that the amplitude of the P2 component differentiated monkey and human faces, the P2 latency differentiated orientation, and the N300/400 differentiated familiarity. Interestingly, the 9-month old infants were also processing species, orientation, and familiarity across several components.

In summary, it appears that early experience with certain types of faces may influence later processing. Moreover, the kinds of faces (different races, different species) present in one's environment during development may influence the formation and specificity of the face-processing system.

Configural Versus Featural Processing

A distinction exists between featural and configural information contained within a face (Diamond and Carey 1977). *Featural* information refers to individual face elements (such as the eyes or mouth), and *configural* information refers to the spatial layout of these elements within the face (Freire and Lee 2001). These sources of information are not mutually exclusive; changes in features necessitate a change in the configural information and changes in configurations involve a concomitant change in the individual features (Tanaka and Sengco 1997). Humans' reliance on configural information in the recognition and processing of faces is demonstrated when faces are inverted (Yin 1969) and also when features of inverted faces are upright (Thompson 1980). Inversion tends to impair recognition of faces more than objects. This effect was first reported by Yin (1969), who found that inversion disrupts the configural processing of a facial stimulus. Yin further reported that children younger than 10 years discriminate unfamiliar upright faces as accurately as unfamiliar inverted faces, whereas adults and older children are impaired in the unfamiliar inverted condition. Thus, with unfamiliar faces, children seem to be better than adults at processing inverted faces compared with upright faces. Farah et al. (1995) contended that faces are represented as holistic units, whereas objects can be broken down into separable parts. Inverting a face presumably causes a disruption in this configural or holistic processing and thus causes decrements in facial information processing such as impaired recognition and delayed reaction time (Freire et al. 2000).

One way to investigate the development of featural and configural processing is to determine where infants and children fixate on faces, what features they look at more than others (if any), and how this changes with development. Maurer and Salapatek (1976) conducted the only study to date that investigates infants' eye fixations while they view faces. They found that 1-month-old infants fixated away from the face for most of the time but that 2-month-old infants fixated on the faces, looking more at specific features, especially internal features and the eyes.

Developmental changes in the processing of featural and configural face information also have been investigated in 9-year-old patients with bilateral congenital cataracts removed between age 2 and 6 months (Le Grand et al. 2001). Results of this study indicated that even after 9 years of normal visual processing, configural face processing was disrupted in these patients. In this investigation, experimenters varied featural and configural information in facial stimuli by slightly changing this information (placing eyes further apart vs. replacing individual features, such as eyes). They found that these patients were impaired in detecting changes in configural but not featural information compared with a typically developing control group. The authors concluded that visual experience with faces early in development (within the first 6 months) is necessary for normal development of configural face processing. Consistent with previous research, these findings suggest that configural and featural information may be developmentally dissociable and that a shift may occur from featural to configural processing during a "period of opportunity" sometime during the first 6 months of life. Furthermore, the authors asserted that because typically developing newborns have poor visual acuity, the visual cortex is only exposed to low-spatial-frequency visual information (outer contours and general location of features). Thus, if infants are deprived of low-spatial-frequency visual information during this period, later configural processing may be impaired.

ERPs also have been used to investigate the neural changes associated with face and eye processing in children ages 4–15 years (Taylor et al. 2001). Children were presented with upright and inverted faces and eyes to determine whether they were using featural or configural information while processing faces. The N170 response was much greater in amplitude and shorter in latency to eyes than to faces in children. These data indicate that early processing of eyes may be functional before the processing of whole faces. Furthermore, the cortical areas involved in processing eyes and faces may be somewhat distinct in development.

Facial Expression and Emotion Processing

It is difficult to study the development of face processing and the mechanisms involved in this development without a discussion of the emotionally salient and highly dynamic information that is provided in the face. Indeed, human faces contain a preponderance of significant information, necessary for social communication. For example, familiarity, emotion expression, congruent dynamic information (e.g., lip movement synchronized with voice), and direction of gaze can all be gleaned from very brief exposures to static and dynamic images of faces. Some researchers have studied what they call the *still-face effect* and have found that infants attend more and show more positive affect to dynamic displays of faces than to still faces (e.g., D'Entremont and Muir 1997). Furthermore, in a recent series of studies, Bahrick et al. (2002) suggested that early in infancy, socially contingent and dynamic information may be so important that facial identity is ignored during the dynamic phases of face-to-face interactions. Thus, it is important to point out that infants' learning about faces is probably not completely dissociable from learning about emotional expressions or dynamic contingencies. Furthermore, whatever the mechanisms are that are involved in the development of face processing, it is likely that dynamic and emotionally salient information plays a major role in their development.

Evidence that the ability to recognize emotional expressions needs little experience to develop is based on research with visual paired comparison and habituation procedures that showed that newborns (by age 36 hours) are able to discriminate (based on increases in looking time) between different types of facial expressions (Field et al. 1982). Several investigations with older infants found inconsistencies in the types of emotions infants are able to discriminate. For example, 3-month-old infants are able to discriminate (by dishabituating) smiling from frowning faces (Barrera and Maurer 1981) but not sad faces from happy faces or surprised faces (Young-Browne et al. 1977). Furthermore, 7-month-old infants will show a looking preference for fearful faces over happy faces (Nelson and Dolgin 1985) and can discriminate happy from fearful in a habituation test but only if they first habituate to happy faces (Nelson et al. 1979). Therefore, it is apparent that in the first year of life, infants are able to show some discrimination of emotions, but this discrimination has not yet reached adultlike maturity (for review, see M. de Haan and Nelson 1998; Nelson and de Haan 1996).

Investigations of the neural underpinnings of the development of emotion processing suggest that infants as young as 7 months are able to differentiate between static pictures of some emotions (Nelson and de Haan 1996). ERPs were recorded from 7-month-old infants while they viewed pictures of happy and fearful expressions in one experiment and angry and fearful expressions in another. Results indicated electrophysiological differentiation between happy and fearful expressions but not between angry and fearful expressions at age 7 months. As stated earlier, the methods typically used to test discrimination of expressions early in development involve viewing static pictures of faces. The use of a more dynamic and intermodal display of emotional expressions indicated that 7-month-old infants were able to discriminate happy and angry expressions by just motion information alone, suggesting that actually viewing the face may not be a necessary component in this type of perception (Soken and Pick 1992). This study illustrates the inextricably tied nature of face and emotion recognition but leaves us wondering whether face recognition, in general, is mediated by mechanisms different from those involved in emotion recognition—or whether emotion recognition is simply an extension of the face recognition system. This question is related to Haxby and colleagues' (2000) notion that emotion information is part of an extended face-processing system (subserved by the amygdala), suggesting that emotion information may indeed be processed separately from the early perception of faces.

Although evidence is limited regarding the neurobiology of the development of emotion expression processing (especially with infants), several adult investigations have studied the timing and underlying neural substrates of such processing (Eimer and Holmes 2002; Pizzagalli et al. 2002). Data from ERP studies suggest that information about the face may be processed separately from information about emotion or affective judgment (Eimer and Holmes 2002; Pizzagalli et al. 2002). Early perceptual ERP components have been found to process affect information before identity information (Pizzagalli et al. 2002). These data suggest that affect processing may play an important role in the structural encoding and identification of faces. It will be important to study the development of the morphology of these early affective-based responses because it may shed light on the mechanisms involved in face and emotion processing. For example, if infants and children are processing emotion information before they process identity, the emotional information in the face may be a big contributor to the developing specificity of face processing.

The amygdala is thought to be involved in the evaluation of emotionally significant stimuli (LeDoux 1996). Emotion face processing has been investigated with fMRI in both typically developing and non–typically developing populations (Baird et al. 1999; Thomas et al. 2001). In adults, the presentation of fearful faces increases activation in the left amygdala compared with the presentation of neutral faces (Thomas et al. 2001). Children (11 years old), in contrast, show greater amygdala activation to neutral compared with fearful faces (Thomas et al. 2001). The authors suggested that this effect may be due to the increased ambiguity (leading to increased vigilance) that a neutral face elicits. Furthermore, the authors asserted that neutral faces may not yet indicate neutrality, and children may therefore be trying to interpret the meaning of the neutral faces, thus increasing vigilance. In contrast to the previous findings, Baird et al. (1999) found that the pattern of response in adolescents and adults was similar—the amygdala had greater activation to fearful compared with neutral faces. Further investigations are needed to replicate these data. Indeed, further research investigating the developmental neurobiology of emotion processing is needed to elucidate the behavioral and neural correlates of this socially relevant system.

Face Processing in Atypically Developing Populations

The study of typical development often can be informed by the study of children who deviate from a normal trajectory. Such is the case with face processing, in which studying children with known impairments in this ability may shed light on how face processing operates in typically developing children. In this section, we focus on both adult and developmental investigations of individuals with prosopagnosia and individuals with autism.

Prosopagnosia

As mentioned earlier, the special nature of face processing compared with other types of visual processing originates from reports of patients who are reportedly unable to recognize familiar faces while maintaining the ability to recognize and identify objects. Patients with this deficit have a syndrome called *prosopagnosia* (De Renzi 1986). This impairment is often accompanied by focal bilateral (usually) damage to the ventral occipitotemporal and temporal cortices (Damasio et al. 1982). For example, patient LH (reviewed by Farah 1996) had damage to an area within the occipitotemporal cortex and experienced impaired recognition of faces in the absence of impaired object recognition. Interestingly, patients with prosopagnosia have been described as processing faces similar to the way in which they process objects. Whereas adults without prosopagnosia process faces in a holistic manner and thus have impairments recognizing inverted faces, almost no performance decrement is seen when prosopagnosic patients are shown inverted faces compared with upright faces (Farah 1995; Yin 1969). Some individuals with prosopagnosia have been reported to have performance advantages over control subjects without prosopagnosia on inverted face processing (Farah 1995). These patients also have been shown to have an abnormal pattern of activation in the fusiform gyrus (Marotta et al. 2001). These authors report left hemisphere posterior fusiform activation suggesting that these patients are processing stimuli in a more feature-based compared with holistic manner (similar to how objects are processed).

A small number of developmental prosopagnosic cases have been reported. The vast majority of these cases have occurred in individuals who have more general visual processing deficits in addition to difficulties recognizing faces (E.H. de Haan and Campbell 1991; Young and Ellis 1989). However, there is a report of a boy who sustained brain damage at age 1 day, now in late adolescence, who has structural damage to occipitotemporal pathways and impairments similar to those typically reported in adults with prosopagnosia (Farah et al. 2000). These authors suggested that this report may be evidence for an innately specified face-processing system; that is, a system that does not require perceptual experience to develop.

Autism

Children with autism are often reported to have deficits in face-processing abilities (Hobson et al. 1988; Kanner 1942; Langdell 1978; Marcus and Nelson 2001). Although a deficit in face processing is not a defining feature of autism, the kinds of impairments these children experience early in development may be a helpful indicator of future social or emotional impairments (Marcus and Nelson 2001). Indeed, children with autism are not proficient at using faces to determine identity. Individuals with autism tend to make little eye contact and have been described as treating people as if they were objects (Kanner 1942). Langdell (1978) first reported a lack of the typical inversion effect in processing of faces in autistic children. Langdell found that older autistic children performed better than control subjects on an inverted face task. This finding has since been replicated; Hobson and colleagues (1988) found that individuals with autism were better than a control group at an emotion-face picture sorting task when the faces were inverted. Trepagnier (1998) asserted that autism may be caused by a failure to develop orientation to facial cues, which then disrupts perceptual and social information processing. Furthermore, other studies of face processing have found aberrant processing of familiar face matching (Boucher et al. 1998) and memory for faces (Hauck et al. 1999) in individuals with autism.

The findings in the previous paragraph suggest that individuals with autism do not appear to process faces in the same specialized manner as do adults and typically developing children. Recent neuroimaging evidence augments this conclusion. Schultz and colleagues (2000) found decreased activation in the fusiform region in a group with autism and Asperger's disorder and increased activation in the inferior temporal gyrus compared with control subjects. Similar to previous behavioral research, the authors suggested that the group with autism and Asperger's disorder may process faces similar to how they process objects and thus do not have a specialized face-processing system. However, it is indeed plausible that this deficit may be secondary to the disorder, and these individuals may have less exposure to faces because they simply orient less to faces compared with typically developing individuals.

In an earlier study, Osterling and Dawson (1994) reported that impairments in social cognition in children with autism might be due to early impairments in face-processing abilities. In this study, home videotapes of infants' 1-year birthdays were retrospectively analyzed. Results of these analyses indicated that failure to attend to other people's faces was the best discriminator between children with and without autism. Dawson and colleagues (2002) further investigated this apparent face-processing deficit by recorded ERPs in a population of 3- and 4-year-old children with autism. Relative to a typically developing group of children and a group of children with developmental delays, children with autism failed to show electrophysiological differentiation of familiar and unfamiliar faces (mother's face vs. a stranger's face) for the Nc and the P400 and positive slow wave components. However, children with autism did show differentiation between familiar and unfamiliar toys for the Nc and P400 (greater amplitude to unfamiliar objects at both components) (Figure 2–4). These results suggest that children with autism may have face-processing deficits at the cortical level and that these deficits occur in the absence of impairments in object processing. In a second ERP study, McPartland et al. (2001a, 2001b) recorded ERPs from adolescents with high-functioning autism. The results of this study also indicated face-processing impairments relative to an IQ-matched control group. More specifically, the latency to peak response of the N170 component was longer in latency and did not show the typical differences between upright and inverted faces. Furthermore, this component was also right lateralized in control subjects but not in individuals with autism.

Recently, Marcus and Nelson (2001) suggested three possible pathways to deficits seen in face processing in individuals with autism. These possible pathways also can be applied to the development of face-processing deficits in Williams syndrome and Turner's syndrome. They suggested that this face-processing system develops in an experience-expectant manner. First, these def-

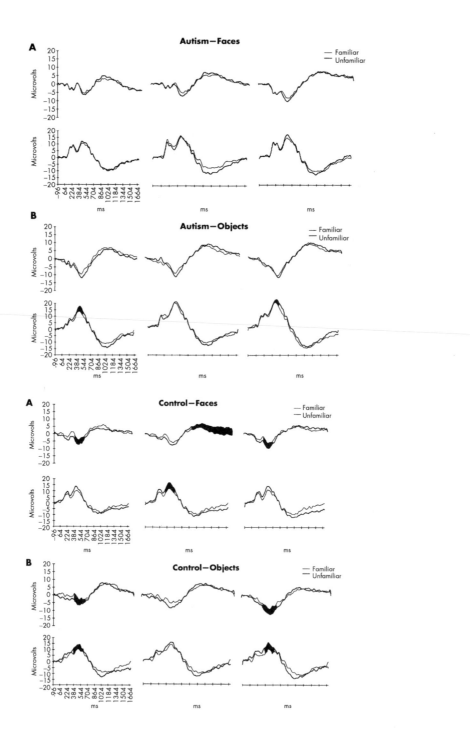

Figure 2–4. Averaged event-related potential waveforms (*opposite page*) at the anterior (top) and posterior (bottom), right hemisphere, midline, and left hemisphere scalp locations for familiar and unfamiliar **A)** *faces* and **B)** *objects* for children with autism spectrum disorders **(top panels)** and children with typical development **(bottom panels).**

Areas in which significant differences were found for familiar versus unfamiliar stimuli are *shaded in black.*

Source. Adapted from Dawson G, Carver L, Meltzoff A, et al.: "Neural Correlates of Face and Object Recognition in Young Children With Autism Spectrum Disorder, Developmental Delay and Typical Development." *Child Development* 73:700–717, 2002. Used with permission.

icits could be accounted for by a lack of the "expected" visual stimuli (faces), which would subsequently influence synaptic pruning (the assumption being that "correct" information in the environment leads to a stabilization of synaptic circuits and a concomitant pruning of unconfirmed and, thus, irrelevant synapses). Second, they suggested that this system may not be receiving normal input; thus, facial stimuli may be present in the environment, but deficits in processing this information, such as social gaze (or failure to recognize important aspects of the stimuli), may fail to sustain normal development of this system. Finally, similar to the second mechanism, they suggested that exposure to a stimulus may not be tantamount to the experience required for that system to develop. For example, children with autism may treat faces as objects, so the development of one specialized system for both objects and faces seems appropriate.

The following question remains: Why are faces and objects being treated similarly in autism? Intuitively, the main difference between objects and faces is the affective or emotional and dynamic information that is portrayed in the face compared with objects. Thus, aberrant interpretation of affective or dynamic stimuli may later influence the development of specialized systems. Indeed, Grelotti and colleagues (2002) suggested that because individuals with autism have reduced social interest, they may fail to develop an expert face-processing system. Grelotti and colleagues reported that adults with autism process faces via more inferior occipitotemporal areas (typically object-processing areas) rather than the expected fusiform area, even in the absence of any structural abnormalities. They further suggested that the damage to the amygdala may influence the apparent lack of social interest because it is likely involved in identifying emotionally salient information. A closer look at the development of facial expression and emotion processing as it relates to the development of general face-processing abilities may be necessary to understand the deficits previously described in the neurodevelopmental disorders as well as the normal development of face processing.

We now turn to a review of current models of the neural bases of the development of face processing, including models based on studies of typically and atypically developing populations.

Developmental Theories of Face Processing

Often, the special nature of face processing is predicated on research reporting that newborns prefer viewing facial stimuli compared with a variety of other complex visual stimuli at birth (Morton and Johnson 1991; Valenza et al. 1996). Some researchers suggest that this initial propensity of newborns to preferentially fixate on facelike stimuli is evidence of an innate or a genetically determined face-processing system (Johnson and Morton 1991; Morton and Johnson 1991). Morton and Johnson proposed a system that they termed *CONSPEC*, which is operational from birth and functions to bias newborns to orient toward stimuli that contain the same basic structure as faces (see recent reviews by M. de Haan et al. 2002a; Nelson 2003). CONSPEC is part of a two-process model proposed to account for the development of face processing (Morton and Johnson 1991). According to this model, CONSPEC is a primitive "kick-start" mechanism that is expressed only when infants first view faces. CONSPEC serves as a guide or foundation to subsequent learning about faces. In this theory, CONSPEC responds exclusively to faces moving in the periphery. The CONSPEC mechanism appears to be functional at birth and thus has been hypothesized to be an innate mechanism that facilitates attention to faces. Moreover, Johnson and colleagues argued that the pulvinar may control the CONSPEC mechanism because of its strong inputs from the superior colliculus, its sensitivity to visual form information, and its highly salient stimuli (Grieve et al. 2000). This orienting response, in effect, biases infants to direct their gaze toward faces. An infant's attention to faces is then held by a more diffuse network of connections that are either strengthened or pruned, based on experience. Thus, CONSPEC does not mediate the fixation of attention; it merely directs the infant's gaze. At approximately age 2 months, CONSPEC is replaced with or "set" by *CONLERN*, an experientially based face-processing mechanism. At this point, face processing becomes more dependent on the learning of faces in the environment surrounding the infant.

Recently, Johnson (2000) updated this two-process model of development and proposed an "interactive specialization" theory to explain why an area of the occipitotemporal cortex called the *fusiform face area* is selectively involved in face processing. This theory suggests that there are developmental changes in the tuning properties and cortical localization of this system that result in specialized activation. Johnson suggested that changes in behavioral specialization will result in changes in cortical localization and that the more finely specified or tuned an area of the cortex becomes, the less likely it will be activated for other types of stimuli. However, the mechanisms responsible for this resultant localization and why this localization occurs preferentially in the occipitotemporal cortex remain unclear. This model suggests that early in development, infants have diffuse cortical activation in response to faces that then becomes more specific with environmental exposure to faces. Subsequently, during the first few months of life, infant face perception is an emergent product of the interaction of early orienting tendencies and the overabundance of facial stimuli in the environment. These early orienting abilities are not the result of an innate cortical face module but instead reflect more primitive innate neural circuitry, involving subcortical areas of the brain. With experience, the diffuse neuronal activation becomes more specific, and the face-processing system thus becomes more specialized.

Developmental experiments investigating early visual preferences in newborns have found that newborns not only have a preference for looking at faces but also have a tendency to prefer looking at patterned stimuli arranged in the configuration of a face but without the details of the face (Simion et al. 2001). Simion and colleagues (2001) suggested an alternative to Morton and Johnson's (1991)

CONSPEC mechanism. They conducted a series of experiments to determine whether newborn preferential orientation to faces compared with other stimuli is because faces are "special" or qualitatively different from nonface stimuli or whether a more general process could account for this preference. The first possibility, the *structural hypothesis,* suggests that an innate face-detecting mechanism exists (CONSPEC). Evidence supporting this hypothesis comes from a study that used visual paired comparison and found that infants prefer to look at a facelike pattern, even when presented together with a stimulus of greater physical salience (e.g., Valenza et al. 1996). Additionally, newborns will preferentially track a moving schematic face over several other nonface patterned stimuli or facelike stimuli with the features scrambled (Johnson et al. 1991; Maurer and Young 1983).

An alternative view to the previously described theories, the *sensory hypothesis,* suggests that faces may not be any different from any other stimuli. According to this hypothesis, faces are subject to filtering by the visual system, and a preference for faces may be due to low-level processes that determine the visibility of the pattern. Easterbrook et al. (1999) reported a study that supports the sensory hypothesis. They found that infants tracked both a schematic face and patterned stimuli containing different arrangements of the same features equally. Based on the evidence for both the structural and the sensory hypotheses, Simion and colleagues (2001) suggested that these two hypotheses may not be mutually exclusive. To examine this further, Simion et al. (2002) reported a series of studies that found that infants prefer to look at stimuli that have a greater number of elements in the upper rather than the lower part of the configuration. This result is supported by research that suggests that the upper part of the visual field is less sensitive than the lower part (in adults) (Previc 1990; Rubin et al. 1996; Sheng et al. 1996); this preference disappears when the outer and inner components of the schematic are congruent. For example, infants look equally at both an upsidedown triangle with two squares at the top and one square at the bottom (facelike) and a right-side-up triangle with two squares at the bottom and one square at the top (nonfacelike). Newborns seem to consistently prefer the stimulus in which both faceness (more components in the upper part of the configuration) and congruency are present compared with stimuli in which only one of the above is present. They suggested that both faceness and the congruence of the inner and outer features combine to create a preference for facelike stimuli. Furthermore, they suggested that infants' preferences for faces at birth are a result of their spontaneous preference (constrained by the visual system) for the structural properties that are embedded in faces. Macchi Cassia et al. (2004) further examined newborns' preferences for faces by using images of natural and scrambled (features rotated but kept in the same general layout and asymmetrical) upright and inverted (inversion was isolated to inner features only) neutral faces while recording fixation time. Results indicated that newborns preferred to look at faces with more features in the upper part of the face regardless of whether they were scrambled (Figure 2–5).

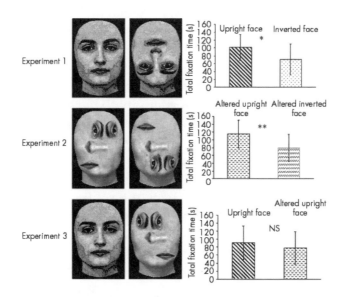

Figure 2–5.   Three pairs of stimuli presented in the three experiments and the total fixation times toward each stimulus in the pairs.

Note.   NS=not significant; *P<0.05; **P<0.001.

Source.   Adapted from Macchi Cassia V, Turati C, Simion F: "Can a Nonspecific Bias Toward Top-Heavy Patterns Explain Newborns' Face Preference?" *Psychological Science* (in press). Used with permission from Blackwell Publishing.

This latter account provides an alternative to CONSPEC: newborn preferences for faces may be a result of the match between structural properties of facelike stimuli and the constraints of the newborn's sensory systems as opposed to an innate subcortical mechanism responsible for directing infants' attention to faces (Simion et al. 2001). Both Morton and Johnson's and Simion and colleagues' accounts explain newborns' initial propensity to fixate on and track faces. Johnson and colleagues (1991) went one step further and proposed an additional mechanism, CONLERN, that guides specialization of face processing. This account does not, however, explain the apparent increasing specificity of the face-processing system or how newborns go on to become "experts" in face processing.

Johnson and Morton's CONLERN mechanism is involved in the maintenance of attention to faces or facelike stimuli. This mechanism takes over for CONSPEC at around age 2 months and is influenced by stimuli in the environment. CONLERN tunes the fusiform face area to become preferentially activated to facial stimuli (M. de Haan et al. 2002a). M. de Haan and colleagues (2002a) argued that this increased specificity of the fusiform face area occurs because of its anatomical location on the ventral visual pathway and high interconnectivity to the hippocampus.

Consistent with adult visual field studies (Ellis and Shepard 1975), lesion sites in adults with prosopagnosia (De Renzi et al. 1994), and adult neuroimaging studies (Gauthier et al. 1999b; Kanwisher et al. 1997), de Schonen and Mathivet (1989, 1990) proposed a model that emphasizes the role of the right hemisphere in the development of face recognition. They found a right hemisphere advantage in face-processing tasks with 4- to 9-month-old infants (de Schonen and Mathivet 1990). They hypothesized that the right hemisphere advantage is a result of the enhanced ability of the right hemisphere to process configural information in early infancy compared with the left hemisphere. Additionally, the right hemisphere is more sensitive to low spatial frequencies (a dominant feature of faces). Because of the competitive nature of the visual system, they hypothesized that experience with faces drives the development of the right hemisphere, which then results in cortical specialization. de Schonen and Mathivet (1989) also pointed out that the left hemisphere does benefit from configural facial information and with time also responds to facial stimuli. Although the difference between configural and featural processing of stimuli during development is compelling, the anatomical basis for a right hemisphere advantage for faces over other low spatial frequency stimuli is unclear. Indeed, most other aspects of the visual system seem to develop in a symmetrical fashion. Furthermore, this theory does not account for why faces drive the development of this specialized visual system over other complex stimuli.

In a recent review, Elgar and Campbell (2001) suggested that investigating the impairments of children with autism, Williams syndrome, and Turner's syndrome will better inform our understanding of normal face processing. Elgar and Campbell suggested that children with autism have face-processing deficits because of aberrant affective and social "drivers." Children with Williams syndrome tend to be highly sociable but have deficits in visual-spatial abilities. Children with Turner's syndrome have mild impairments in social functioning and relatively poor visual-spatial and perceptual-organizational abilities. Elgar and Campbell proposed a model that asserts that two "drivers" are involved in face processing—an affective/social driver and a visual-spatial driver. They suggested that these drivers are interactive and multiplicative in modulating the development of face expertise. They also argued that deficits in the visual-spatial driver may be a result of damage to magnocellular visual projections from the lateral geniculate nucleus to the occipital cortex and then up through the dorsal stream. Compared with the ventral visual pathway, the dorsal visual pathway receives most of the information from magnocellular projections. The ventral visual pathway receives information from both magno- and parvocelluar projections. They suggested that the function of the magnocellular cells (sensitive to high temporal and low spatial frequency and highly responsive to movement) further supports this idea. Elgar and Campbell also suggested that because the superior temporal sulcus receives information from both the ventral and the dorsal streams, the superior temporal sulcus may be preferentially involved in processing dynamic facial information. They suggested that the affective/social driver is mediated by the ventromedial parts of the inferior frontal cortex, which plays a key role in moderating activity flowing to the cortex from the amygdala and thalamus, among other subcortical structures.

Nelson (1993, 2001, 2003) proposed a model of the development of face perception that accounts for how humans become experts at perceiving and processing facial information. This model suggests that infants mold their face-processing system based on the visual experiences they encounter. Nelson's model of the development of face perception draws an analogy to speech perception, in that, similar to speech perception, there appears to be a potential for cortical specialization that is dependent on experience (for review, see Kuhl 1993, 1997). Among other investigators, Kuhl and colleagues have reported that before age 6–8 months, infants are able to discriminate between a wide range of phonemes, or basic sound units. This ability tends to narrow with repeated experience to phonemes in one's native language and a lack of experience with phonemes outside one's own language (Cheour et al. 1998; Kuhl et al. 1997). Nelson (2001, 2003) suggested that this type of "perceptual narrowing" also may occur in face perception. Moreover, he asserted that early in development, humans may have the ability to discriminate between a wide range of faces and facial features and that based on environmental stimulation, or the types of faces infants are exposed to, this system becomes more specific. Thus, with development, the ability to discriminate between faces that one has not had exposure to is not as good as the ability to discriminate between faces one has had experience differentiating. This model of the development of face processing contrasts some of the previously discussed models by proposing a solely experience-expectant and activity-dependent developmental progression (Nelson 2001, 2003). Support for Nelson's (2001, 2003) perceptual narrowing model comes from several adult and developmental investigations, including research on the other-race and other-species effects, the formation of a prototypical face, and the perceptual expertise effect. For example, although further research is needed, it is plausible that the other-race and other-species effects are due to the amount of differential experience infants have with different types of faces while forming an expert face-processing system.

Consistent with this idea, some researchers have suggested that faces are represented as a comparison to a prototype that has been formed through experience. This prototype roughly represents an average of the kinds of faces or features one has seen. Indeed, Rhodes et al. (1993) argued that the coding of faces occurs by making a comparison between the perceived face and a prototype. Thus, the decrement in performance that is seen while processing inverted faces may be due to the difficulties that occur when comparing rotated faces with the prototype. Many models of face recognition (both developmental and adult theories) agree that the brain must store some sort of representation of faces (at many different levels), but they differ as to the form of this representation and how it is compared with other faces already encoded in memory. Support for the development of a "prototype" comes from studies suggesting that infants consistently prefer to view attractive faces when paired with unattractive faces (Langlois et al. 1987; Slater et al. 1998). Attractive faces are seen as more facelike because they more closely match the facial representation or prototype that infants either acquire from their experience of seeing faces or are born with. Johnson and de Haan (2001) assessed infants' ability to extract a prototype from a series of individual faces. They observed that in 3-month-old infants but not 1-month-old infants, the prototypical stimulus was more familiar than the familiar trained face. They suggested that the ability to extract invariances from a set of input faces develops between ages 1 and 3 months.

Gauthier and colleagues suggested that visual areas selective for recognition of faces can be recruited through expertise for nonface objects, such as greebles (or facelike objects), birds, or cars (Gauthier and Tarr 1997; Gauthier et al. 2000). Therefore, without expertise, face perception would be similar to any other kind of object processing (Gauthier and Nelson 2001). The idea of perceptual expertise emphasizes the importance of early and continued visual experience with faces in order for adultlike (expert) face processing to develop. Further research on perceptual expertise supports Nelson's perceptual narrowing theory, but it does not describe the mechanisms involved in the development of this expert system.

Analytical Summary of Theories

Each of these models and interpretations is intriguing; however, there are several unanswered questions, as well as several unfounded assumptions, for which new models of face processing development need to account. None of the above views appears sufficient to explain 1) why this apparent progression from a general to a more specific face-processing system occurs and 2) why specific areas of the cortex are targeted to preferentially process faces. Johnson's interactive perspective attempts to account for some of the above, but the neural and behavioral mechanisms involved in the developmental progression from a genetically or subcortically controlled system to an experience-based system are not well specified. For example, it is unclear why CONSPEC is specific to faces and not to more general complex visual patterns (particularly moving patterns). It is also not clear why both systems are not functional at birth or how CONLERN "takes over" for CONSPEC. Additionally, the development of a specialized cortical area devoted to processing only facial stimuli is puzzling. Is there any evidence, as de Schonen and colleagues asserted, that the neural tissue in the right hemisphere or, more specifically, in the right fusiform area is more appropriate for processing faces compared with objects? If so, how does CONLERN, or whatever mechanisms are responsible for translating this information during development, know which cortical area(s) should become specialized for faces? Johnson postulated an initial genetic mechanism, but it is still unclear why this mechanism is necessary. For example, given that newborns are inundated with facial information from the moment they are born, it is not clear why a genetic mechanism needs to be postulated to account for early facial preferences. Moreover, it is unclear whether CONLERN is influenced by changes in cortical specialization that result in changes in behavior or whether changes in behavior result in cortical specialization.

Nelson's model (2001, 2003) has support from fields spanning developmental and cognitive science, but the mechanisms involved in this increasing specialization are not yet well understood. For example, it is unclear what narrows, what parts of the brain are involved in controlling this narrowing, and whether such narrowing is specific to faces (and speech). Also, several questions remain unanswered regarding the evidence that supports this model. For example, the specificity and malleability of the formation of a prototype are not well specified. It is plausible to imagine a system that forms a prototype through experience with different types of features and faces and the simultaneous development of configural processing, but further investigations are needed to verify this hypothesis and determine the underlying neurobiology of configural and featural processing as well as prototype formation. The effects of the formation of a prototype may result in the other-race and other-species biases reported earlier in this chapter. Another interesting question is whether the other-race effect is apparent in infants and/or young children. Or, based on Nelson's model, do infants and/or young children have an enhanced ability, compared with adults, to perceive and differentiate novel types of features and faces? Furthermore, it may be interesting to examine age effects. For example, do 7-year-old children have a 7-year-old prototype that allows them to process 7-year-old faces more rapidly than faces of other ages?

Notably, only one of the previously described models accounts for the role of the highly dynamic and emotionally salient information provided in faces that newborns encounter just a few seconds after birth and for the rest of their lives. Elgar and Campbell give a provocative account of the development of face processing, based on research with individuals who have developmental disorders, and suggest a role for the influence of socioemotional information. Although rather intriguing, further research needs to be conducted to validate the proposed neuroanatomical pathways and behavioral correlates to these pathways. Additionally, Elgar and Campbell's model does not account for the development of expertise or the increasingly specific processing of faces across development and why their proposed drivers only pick up the dynamics of face information.

Conclusion

In summary, the study of the developmental neurobiology of face processing is still in its infancy. Despite the relatively large body of literature on adult face processing as well as the behavioral correlates of the development of face processing, relatively little is known about the neural correlates that mediate the development of this system. The evidence presented in this chapter largely suggests that the development of face processing can be characterized as an experience-expectant process, influenced by many different factors. Moreover, the development of this perceptual ability may occur during a "period of opportunity" when visual face information present in the environment molds the specificity of this system. Although it is unclear what kind of visual information is necessary to shape this system, it is likely a combination of many factors, including preferences or limitations of the newborn visual system, basic perceptual information about faces (symmetry; more features in the upper half), social and dynamic information, familiarity, and simply because we see so many faces every day (possibly leading to expertise).

As summarized earlier, neuroimaging techniques have recently begun to be used to study the development of face processing. Studies that use these techniques have not only begun to elucidate the neural machinery involved in the development of this system but also have begun to shed light on the neural mechanisms involved in mature face processing. Future advances in imaging technologies that allow for noninvasive investigations in both developmental and disordered populations will greatly benefit the study of face processing. Moreover, collaborative efforts that focus on the acquisition and development of face processing across the life span, using both behavioral and neuroscientific methods, may provide more informative models and theories related to this perceptual ability. More specifically, a complete theory of face processing must characterize face processing from start to finish and must account for the mechanisms that influence the behavioral and cortical specificity in the formation of this system.

References

Bahrick LE, Gogate LJ, Ruiz I: Attention and memory for faces and actions in infancy: the salience of actions over faces in dynamic events. Child Dev 6:1629–1643, 2002

Baird AA, Gruber SA, Fein DA, et al: Functional magnetic resonance imaging and facial affect recognition in children and adolescents. J Am Acad Child Adolesc Psychiatry 38:195–199, 1999

Barrera ME, Maurer D: The perception of facial expressions by the three-month old. Child Dev 52:203–206, 1981

Boucher J, Lewis V, Collis G: Familiar face and voice matching and recognition in children with autism. J Child Psychol Psychiatry 39:171–181, 1998

Brigham J, Barkowitz P: Do "they all look alike?" The effect of race, sex, experience and attitudes on the ability to recognize faces. J Appl Soc Psychol 8:306–318, 1978

Brigham J, Malpass R: The role of experience and contact in the recognition of own- and other-race persons. J Soc Issues 41:139–155, 1985

Carmel D, Bentin S: Domain specificity versus expertise: factors influencing distinct processing of faces. Cognition 83:1–29, 2002

Carver LJ, Dawson G, Panagiotides H, et al: Age-related differences in neural correlates of face recognition during the toddler and preschool years. Dev Psychobiol 42:148–159, 2003

Chance JE, Turner AL, Goldstein AG: Development of differential recognition for own- and other-race faces. J Psychol 112:29–37, 1982

Cheour M, Ceponiene R, Lehtokoski A, et al: Development of language-specific phoneme representations in the infant brain. Nat Neurosci 1:351–353, 1998

D'Entremont B, Muir DW: Five-month-olds' attention and affective responses to still faced emotional expressions. Infant Behavior and Development 20:563–568, 1997

Damasio AR, Damasio HC, Van Hoesen GW: Prosopagnosia: anatomic basis and behavioral mechanisms. Neurology 4:1–15, 1982

Dawson G, Carver L, Meltzoff A, et al: Neural correlates of face and object recognition in young children with autism spectrum disorder, developmental delay and typical development. Child Dev 73:700–717, 2002

DeBoer T, Scott LS, Nelson CA: Event-related potentials in developmental populations, in Event-Related Potentials: A Methods Handbook. Edited by Handy TC. MA, MIT Press (in press) de Haan EH, Campbell R: A fifteen year follow-up case of developmental prosopagnosia. Cortex 27:489–509, 1991

de Haan M, Nelson CA: Recognition of the mother's face by 6-month-old infants: a neurobehavioral study. Child Dev 68:187–210, 1997

de Haan M, Nelson CA: Discrimination and categorization of facial expressions of emotion during infancy, in Perceptual Development: Visual, Auditory, and Language Perception in Infancy. Edited by Slater AM. London, University College London Press, 1998, pp 287–309

de Haan M, Nelson CA: Electrocortical correlates of face and object recognition by 6-month-old infants. Dev Psychol 35:187–210, 1999

de Haan M, Thomas KM: Application of ERP and fMRI techniques to developmental science. Developmental Science 5:335–343, 2002

de Haan M, Humphreys K, Johnson MH: Developing a brain specialized for face perception: a converging methods approach. Dev Psychobiol 40:200–212, 2002a

de Haan M, Pascalis O, Johnson MH: Specialization of neural mechanisms underlying face recognition in human infants. J Cogn Neurosci 12:199–209, 2002b

De Renzi E: Current issues in prosopagnosia, in Aspects of Face Processing. Edited by Ellis HD, Jeeves MD, Newcombe F, et al. Dordrecht, The Netherlands, Nijhoff, 1986, pp 243–252

De Renzi E, Perani D, Carlesimo GA, et al: Prosopagnosia can be associated with damage confined to the right hemisphere—an MRI and PET study and review of the literature. Neuropsychologia 32:893–902, 1994

de Schonen S, Mathivet E: First come, first served: a scenario about the development of hemispheric specialization in face recognition during infancy. European Bulletin of Cognitive Psychology 9:3–44, 1989

de Schonen S, Mathivet E: Hemispheric asymmetry in a face discrimination task in infants. Child Dev 61:1192–1205, 1990

Diamond R, Carey S: Developmental changes in the representation of faces. J Exp Child Psychol 86:55–87, 1977

Easterbrook MA, Kisilevsky BS, Hains SMJ, et al: Faceness or complexity: evidence from newborn visual tracking of facelike stimuli. Infant Behavior and Development 22:17–35, 1999

Eimer M, Holmes A: An ERP study on the time course of emotional face processing. Neuroreport 13:427–431, 2002

Elgar R, Campbell R: The development of face-identification skills: what lies behind the face module? Infant and Child Development 10:25–30, 2001

Ellis HD, Shepard JW: Recognition of upright and inverted faces presented in the left and right visual fields. Cortex 11:3–7, 1975

Fallshore M, Scholler JW: Verbal vulnerability of perceptual expertise. J Exp Psychol Learn Mem Cogn 21:1608–1623, 1995

Farah MJ: Face perception and within-category discrimination in prosopagnosia. Neuropsychologia 33:661–674, 1995

Farah MJ: Is face recognition 'special'? Evidence from neuropsychology. Behav Brain Res 76:181–189, 1996

Farah MJ, Wilson KD, Drain M, et al: The inverted face inversion effect in prosopagnosia: evidence for mandatory, face-specific perceptual mechanisms. Vision Res 35:2089–2093, 1995

Farah MJ, Rabinowitz C, Quinn GE, et al: Early commitment of neural substrates for face recognition. Cognitive Neuropsychology 17:117–123, 2000

Field TM, Woodson RW, Greenberg R, et al: Discrimination and imitation of facial expressions by neonates. Science 218:179–181, 1982

Freire A, Lee K, Symons LA: The face-inversion effect as a deficit in the encoding of configural information: direct evidence. Perception 29:159–170, 2000

Freire A, Lee K: Face recognition in 4- to 7-year-olds: processing of configural, featural, and paraphernalia information. J Exp Child Psychol 80:347–371, 2001

Furl N, Phillips JP, O'Toole AJ: Face recognition algorithms and the other-race effect: computational mechanisms for a developmental contact hypothesis. Cognitive Science 96:1–19, 2002

Gauthier I, Nelson CA: The development of face expertise. Curr Opin Neurobiol 11:219–224, 2001

Gauthier I, Tarr MJ: Becoming a "Greeble" expert: exploring mechanisms for face recognition. Vision Res 37:1673–1682, 1997

Gauthier I, Williams P, Tarr MJ, et al: Training 'greeble' experts: a framework for studying expert object recognition processes. Vision Res 38:2401–2428, 1998

Gauthier I, Behrmann M, Tarr MJ: Can face recognition really be dissociated from object recognition? J Cogn Neurosci 11:349–370, 1999a

Gauthier I, Tarr MJ, Anderson AW, et al: Activation of the middle fusiform 'face area' increases with expertise in recognizing novel objects. Nat Neurosci 2:568–573, 1999b

Gauthier I, Skudlarski P, Gore JC, et al: Expertise for cars and birds recruits brain areas involved in face recognition. Nat Neurosci 3:191–197, 2000

Golby AJ, Gabrieli JDE, Chiao JY, et al: Differential responses in the fusiform region to same-race and other-race faces. Nat Neurosci 4:845–850, 2001

Grelotti DJ, Gauthier I, Schultz RT: Social interest and the development of cortical face specialization: what autism teaches us about face processing. Dev Psychobiol 40:213–225, 2002

Grieve KL, Acuna C, Cudeiro J: The primate pulvinar nuclei: vision and action. Trends Neurosci 23:35–39, 2000

Gross CG, Bender DB, Rocha-Miranda CE: Visual receptive fields of neurons in inferotemporal cortex of the monkey. Science 166:1303–1306, 1969

Gross CG, Rocha-Miranda CE, Bender DB: Visual properties of neurons in inferotemporal cortex of the macaque. J Neurophysiol 35:96–111, 1972

Halit H, de Haan M, Johnson MH: Cortical specialization for face processing: face-sensitive event-related potential components in 3- and 12-month-old infants. Neuroimage 19:1180–1193, 2003

Hauck M, Fein D, Maltby N, et al: Memory for faces in children with autism. Child Neuropsychology 4:187–198, 1999

Haxby JV, Hoffman EA, Gobbini MI: The distributed human neural system for face perception. Trends Neurosci 4:223–233, 2000

Haxby JV, Gobbini MI, Furey ML, et al: Distributed and overlapping representations of faces and objects in ventral temporal cortex. Science 293:2425–2430, 2001

Hobson RP, Ouston J, Lee A: What's in a face? The case of autism. Br J Psychol 79:441–453, 1988

Johnson MH: Functional brain development in infants: elements of an interactive specialization framework. Child Dev 71:74–81, 2000

Johnson MH, de Haan M: Developing cortical specialization for visual-cognitive function: the case of face recognition, in Mechanisms of Cognitive Development: Behavioral and Neural Perspectives. Edited by McClelland JL, Siegler RS. Mahwah, NJ, Lawrence Erlbaum, 2001, pp 253–270

Johnson MH, Morton J: Biology and Cognitive Development: The Case of Face Recognition. Oxford, England, Blackwell, 1991

Johnson MH, Dziurawiec S, Ellis H, et al: Newborns' preferential tracking of face-like stimuli and its subsequent decline. Cognition 40:1–19, 1991

Kanner L: Autistic disturbances of affective contact. Nerv Child 2:217–250, 1942

Kanwisher N, McDermott J, Chun MM: The fusiform face area: a module in human extrastriate cortex specialized for face perception. J Neurosci 17:4302–4311, 1997

Kuhl PK: Innate predispositions and the effects of experience in speech perception: the native language magnet theory, in Developmental Neurocognition: Speech and Face Processing in the First Year of Life. Edited by de Boysson-Bardies B, de Schonen S, Jusczyk P, et al. Hinghan, MA, Kluwer Academic Press, 1993, pp 259–274

Kuhl PK, Andruski JE, Chistovich IA, et al: Cross-language analysis of phonetic units in language addressed to infants. Science 277:684–686, 1997

Langdell T: Recognition of faces: an approach to the study of autism. British Journal of Child Psychology and Psychiatry 19:255–268, 1978

Langlois JH, Roggman LA, Casey RJ, et al: Infant preferences for attractive faces: rudiments of a stereotype? Dev Psychol 23:363–369, 1987

LeDoux JE: The Emotional Brain. New York, Simon & Schuster, 1996

Le Grand R, Mondloch CJ, Maurer D, et al: Neuroperception: early visual experience and face processing (letter). Nature 410:890, 2001

Macchi Cassia V, Turati C, Simion F: Can a non-specific bias toward top-heavy patterns explain newborns' face preference? Psychol Sci (in press)

Malpass RS, Kravitz J: Recognition for faces of own and other race. J Pers Soc Psychol 13:330–334, 1969

Marcus D, Nelson CA: Neural bases and development of face recognition in autism. CNS Spectr 6:36–59, 2001

Marotta JJ, Genovese CR, Behrmann M: A functional MRI study of face recognition in patients with prosopagnosia. Neuroreport 12:1581–1587, 2001

Maurer D, Salapatek P: Developmental changes in the scanning of faces by young children. Child Dev 47:523–537, 1976

Maurer D, Young R: Newborns' following of natural and distorted arrangements of facial features. Infant Behavior and Development 6:127–131, 1983

McPartland J, Dawson G, Carver L, et al: Neural correlates of face perception in autism. Poster presented at the meeting of the Society for Research in Child Development, Minneapolis, MN, April 2001a

McPartland J, Dawson G, Carver L, et al: Neural correlates of face perception in individuals with autism spectrum disorder. Poster presented at the International Meeting for Autism Research, San Diego, CA, November 2001b

Morton J, Johnson MH: CONSPEC and CONLERN: a two-process theory of infant face recognition. Psychological Press 98:164–181, 1991

Nelson CA: The recognition of facial expressions in infancy: behavioral and electrophysiological correlates, in Developmental Neurocognition: Speech and Face Processing in the First Year of Life. Edited by de Boysson-Bardies B, de Schonen S, Jusczyk P, et al. Hinghan, MA, Kluwer Academic Press, 1993, pp 187–193

Nelson CA: Neural correlates of recognition memory in the first postnatal year of life, in Human Behavior and the Developing Brain. Edited by Dawson G, Fischer K. New York, Guilford, 1994, pp 269–313

Nelson CA: The development and neural bases of face recognition. Infant and Child Development 10:3–18, 2001

Nelson CA: The development of face recognition reflects an experience-expectant and activity dependent process, in The Development of Face Processing in Infancy and Early Childhood: Current Perspectives. Edited by Pascalis O, Slater A. New York, Nova Science Publishers, 2003, pp 79–97

Nelson CA, Bloom FE: Child development and neuroscience. Child Dev 68:970–987, 1997

Nelson CA, Collins PF: Event-related potential and looking time analysis of infants' responses to familiar and novel events: implications for visual recognition memory. Dev Psychol 27:50–58, 1991

Nelson CA, de Haan M: A neurobehavioral approach to the recognition of facial expressions in infancy, in The Psychology of Facial Expression. Edited by Russell JA. Cambridge, MA, Cambridge University Press, 1996, pp 176–204

Nelson CA, Dolgin K: The generalized discrimination of facial expressions by 7-month-old infants. Child Dev 56:58–61, 1985

Nelson CA, Monk C: The use of event-related potentials in the study of cognitive development, in Handbook of Developmental Cognitive Neuroscience. Edited by Nelson CA, Luciana M. Cambridge, Massachusetts Institute of Technology Press, 2001, pp 125–136

Nelson CA, Morse PA, Leavitt LA: Recognition of facial expressions by seven-month-old infants. Child Dev 50:1239–1242, 1979

Nelson CA, Bloom FE, Cameron J, et al: An integrative, multidisciplinary approach to the study of brain-behavior relations in the context of typical and atypical development. Dev Psychopathol 14:499–520, 2002

Osterling J, Dawson G: Early recognition of children with autism: a study of first birthday home videotapes. J Autism Dev Disord 24:247–257, 1994

O'Toole AJ, Deffenbacher KA, Valentin D, et al: Structural aspects of face recognition and the other-race effect. Mem Cognit 22:208–224, 1994

Pascalis O, Bachevalier J: Face recognition in primates: a cross-species study. Behav Processes 43:87–96, 1998

Pascalis O, de Schonen S: Recognition memory in 3- to 4-day-old human neonates. Neuroreport 5:1721–1724, 1994

Pascalis O, de Schonen S, Morton J, et al: Mother's face recognition by neonates: a replication and extension. Infant Behavior and Development 18:79–95, 1995

Pascalis O, Demont E, de Haan M, et al: Recognition of faces of different species: a developmental study between 5 and 8 years of age. Infant and Child Development 10:39–45, 2001

Pascalis O, de Haan M, Nelson CA: Is face processing species-specific during the first year of life? Science 296:1321–1323, 2002

Passarotti AM, Paul BM, Bussiere JR, et al: The development of face and location processing: an fMRI study. Developmental Science 6:100–117, 2003

Perrett DI, Rolls ET, Caan W: Visual neurons responsive to faces in the monkey temporal cortex. Experimental Brain Research 47:329–342, 1982

Perrett DI, Mistlin AJ, Chitty AJ: Visual neurons responsive to faces. Trends Neurosci 10:358–364, 1987

Pizzagalli DA, Lehmann D, Hendrick AM, et al: Affective judgments of faces modulate early activity (~160 ms) within the fusiform gyri. Neuroimage 16:663–677, 2002

Previc FH: Functional specialization in the lower and upper visual field in humans: its ecological origins and neurophysiological implications. Behav Brain Sci 13:519–575, 1990

Rhodes G, Brake D, Atkinson AP: What's lost in inverted faces? Cognition 47:25–57, 1993

Rubin N, Nakayama K, Shapley R: Enhanced perception of illusory contours in the lower versus upper visual hemifield. Science 271:651–653, 1996

Schultz RT, Gauthier I, Klin A, et al: Abnormal ventral temporal cortical activity during face discrimination among individuals with autism and Asperger syndrome. Arch Gen Psychiatry 57:331–340, 2000

Scott LS, Nelson CA: Increasing specificity in face processing: a developmental ERP study. Poster presented at Cognitive Neuroscience Society Annual Meeting, New York, NY, March 2003

Sheng H, Cavanagh P, Intriligator J: Attentional resolution and the locus of visual awareness. Nature 383:334–337, 1996

Simion F, Macchi Cassia V, Turati C, et al: The origins of face perception: specific versus non-specific mechanisms. Infant and Child Development 10:59–65, 2001

Simion F, Valenza E, Macchi Cassia V, et al: Newborns' preference for up-down asymmetrical configurations. Developmental Science 5:427–434, 2002

Slater A, Von der Schulenburg C, Brown E, et al: Newborn infants prefer attractive faces. Infant Behavior and Development 21:345–354, 1998

Soken NH, Pick A: Intermodal perception of happy and angry expressive behaviors by seven-month-old infants. Child Dev 63:787–795, 1992

Tanaka JW, Sengco JA: Features and their configuration in face recognition. Mem Cognit 25:583–592, 1997

Taylor MJ, Edmonds GE, McCarthy G, et al: Eyes first! Eye processing develops before face processing in children. Neuroreport 12:1671–1676, 2001

Thomas K, Drevets WC, Whalen PJ, et al: Amygdala response to facial expressions in children and adults. Biol Psychiatry 49:309–316, 2001

Thompson P: Margaret Thatcher: a new illusion. Perception 9:483–484, 1980

Trepagnier C: Autism etiology: a face-processing perspective. Brain Cogn 37:158–160, 1998

Valenza E, Simion F, Cassia VM, et al: Face preference at birth. J Exp Psychol Hum Percept Perform 22:892–903, 1996

Yin RK: Looking at upside-down faces. J Exp Psychol Gen 81:141–145, 1969

Young AW, Ellis HD: Childhood prosopagnosia. Brain Cogn 9:16–47, 1989

Young-Browne G, Rosenfeld HM, Horowitz FD: Infant discrimination of facial expressions. Child Dev 48:555–562, 1977

Chapter 3

Developmental Psychobiology of Reading Disability

Bruce D. McCandliss, Ph.D.
Michael Wolmetz, B.S.

The acquisition of reading serves as a foundational skill for a great deal of later educational and intellectual development. Most children, over the course of several years of formal education and practice, develop specialized perceptual skills that support the fluent and effortless recognition of visual words. Many, however, do not. Impairment in reading skill development is arguably the most prevalent form of learning disability. Substantial and persistent difficulties in the development of reading skill are estimated to affect approximately 5%–15% of the population in the United States (Rutter 1978; Stanovich 1986). Reading disorder is typically diagnosed as a clinical disorder in DSM-IV-TR (American Psychiatric Association 2000) and characterized by poor reading achievement, quantified by standardized tests of reading accuracy, fluency, and comprehension, that falls substantially below expected levels given an individual's chronological age, measured intelligence, and education.

Like many other clinical disorders considered in this volume, reading disability has been investigated under the framework of developmental psychobiology, which involves understanding the symptoms of clinical disorders that affect mental function by examining the underlying cognitive processes involved, linking these processes to specific brain mechanisms, and characterizing how these factors unfold over the course of development. In reviewing this research, in this chapter, we first examine cognitive processes that have been proposed to play a causal role in the complex symptoms of reading impairments. We then review evidence linking core cognitive deficits in reading disability to differences in brain function and structure that exist between individuals with and without reading disability. Beginning with neuroimaging research comparing adults with and without reading disorder, we examine common brain regions implicated at the end state of reading development. Next, we examine the developmental course of these cognitive and neurobiological factors across several recent developmental neuroimaging studies contrasting children with and without reading disability. Several recent studies have combined neuroimaging with cognitive training studies to examine links between improvements in cognitive skills and the accompanying changes in neurobiological processes associated with reading disability. Such studies indicate the potential plasticity (i.e., capacity for change) of cortical circuitry linked to reading skills and provide a potential framework for future research to examine causal relations between intervention efforts and changes in functional brain activity.

Cognitive Deficits in Reading Disability

A significant body of cognitive research has focused on understanding reading disability as a manifestation of more fundamental cognitive deficits that are intrinsic to a child's basic abilities. The past several decades of cognitive research in reading development have provided converging evidence in support of the hypothesis that cognitive deficits in phonological processing abilities play a primary causal role in the development of reading disabilities. Reading disability (i.e., developmental dyslexia) has been systematically linked to impaired performance in several specific tasks that tap phonological processes, such as phonological awareness (the ability to access and flexibly use the speech sounds within syllables, as in rhyming tasks and phoneme blending tasks) (e.g., Bradley and Bryant 1985; Manis et al. 1993), verbal short-term memory (e.g., Jorm 1983; Paulesu et al. 2001; Torgesen et al. 1988), and rapid naming of common visual stimuli (Denkla and Rudel 1976; Wolf 1984). Direct links between various phonological processing deficits and reading disorder have been shown in adults (Pennington et al. 1990) as well as children (National Reading Panel 2000). These phonological processing deficits have been theorized to have a causal influence on the development of reading skill by affecting the early phases of literacy acquisition (Bradley and Bryant 1983). Evidence in support of this core phonological deficit in reading disorder has been surprisingly consistent across two decades of research.

A host of other cognitive deficits have been reported in subsets of dyslexic adults, but with varying degrees of consistency across studies and even less consistency in accounting for variance in reading measures (for recent review, see Ramus 2003). One class of proposed cognitive deficits involves processing rapid temporal information in the auditory modality, with studies suggesting that a primary deficit involving rapid auditory perceptual abilities may underlie previously reported phonological and reading difficulties (Tallal 1980). More contemporary work, however, in both adult dyslexic individuals (Chiappe et al. 2002) and children followed up longitudinally from kindergarten to grade 2 (Share et al. 2002) showed that phonological and reading deficits cannot be reduced to, or predicted by, more basic deficits in processing rapid auditory information. Furthermore, auditory deficits across studies are estimated to appear in approximately 39% of dyslexic individuals and are generally not specific to the processing of rapid temporal information (Ramus 2003).

Other classes of cognitive deficits that might play a critical role in reading disability include perceptual mechanisms in vision involving magnocellular processing pathways (Stein 2001) and cerebellar-motor functions that affect learning, timing, and automaticity (Nicholson et al. 2001). Although evidence from these initial studies links these cognitive deficits to dyslexia, results from several extensive replication efforts have raised concerns about the specificity of visual deficits to the magnocellular system, the prevalence of magnocellular and cerebellar processing deficits in dyslexia, and the relation between the severity of such deficits and actual reading ability (Ramus 2003). One study directly assessed a wide range of cognitive skills in a single well-characterized group of dyslexic adults. Phonological deficits were the only type of difficulty present in nearly every case, and nearly a third of the sample showed no significant signs of sensory or motor deficits (Ramus et al. 2003).

In general, the current state of the literature supports phonological deficits as the dominant core cognitive deficit associated with reading disorder. The influence of other forms of cognitive deficits on reading disorder remains more controversial, in terms of both the relative prevalence and the specific nature by which the proposed cognitive deficit affects the acquisition and skilled performance of reading. In the following section, we examine evidence from neuroimaging studies that seeks to elucidate the relation between phonological processes and reading disability.

Neuroimaging Studies of Adults With Reading Disability

In vivo brain imaging techniques, such as positron-emission tomography (PET) and functional magnetic resonance imaging (fMRI), have provided an important approach for investigating activity within specific cortical regions and associated cognitive deficits linked to reading disability. Flowers and colleagues (1991) provided perhaps one of the first empirical links between cognitive operations involved in phonological processing and patterns of functional disruption in left posterior cortical activity. Adults with childhood histories of reading disorder performed an auditory spelling task while regional cerebral blood flow was imaged in 16 brain regions via a xenon inhalation imaging method (Flowers et al. 1991). The results showed reduced activity in posterior temporal regions in subjects with reading disorder relative to nonimpaired subjects. The following year, a similar finding was reported in a PET study examining phonological processing impairment with a similar auditory spelling test (Rumsey et al. 1992). This finding of less left posterior temporal responsiveness to phonologically demanding tasks in adults with dyslexia relative to nonimpaired readers became a central focus of this literature.

Since these initial studies, advances in brain imaging methodology and analysis have provided the opportunity to perform more comprehensive studies of the biological substrates of reading disorder (for recent review, see McCandliss and Noble 2003). For example, contemporary imaging methods provide whole brain imaging with voxel-by-voxel–analysis rather than region-of-interest analysis. Magnetoencephalography (MEG) studies provide additional information about the time course of activity in various regions on a millisecond timescale. Table 3–1 summarizes the key findings of the neuroimaging studies that involve direct comparisons between adults with reading disorder and nonimpaired adults performing cognitive tasks related to reading or phonological processes.

Several convergent findings relevant to understanding the neurobiology of reading disability become apparent when reviewing the control results of these studies. First, subjects with reading disorder show reduced activity in left posterior regions of temporal cortex, commonly including left superior temporal gyrus, as well as in other neighboring regions such as left angular gyrus and left supramarginal gyrus when performing reading or other phonologically demanding tasks. This central finding is now supported across a wide variety of tasks that target phonological processing regardless of input (auditory words or visual letters) or response modality (i.e., oral pronunciation, button pressing) and suggests that failure to successfully recruit left perisylvian regions when facing phonologically demanding tasks may provide an important neurobiological marker for dyslexia. This result establishes an important connection between findings of core phonological deficits in reading impairments and atypical brain activation patterns associated with phonological processes.

Some effects have been reported in which subjects with reading disorder produced greater activity than did nonimpaired readers in left frontal regions, a pattern hypothesized to reflect alternative strategies that are engaged to compensate for poor phonological skills. Two studies have reported such effects in left frontal regions, specifically within the left inferior frontal gyrus (S.E. Shaywitz et al. 1998) and left insular cortex (Rumsey et al.

Table 3–1. Neuroimaging studies comparing adults with reading disorder and nonimpaired adults performing cognitive tasks related to reading or phonological processes

Authors	Subjects (*n*)	Stimuli	Active task	Control	Type of effect	Group effect	Region
				PET			
Rumsey et al. 1992[a]	NI (14) RD (14)	Auditory word pairs Tones	Rhyme matching: auditory words	Intensity matching: tones	Active>control	NI>RD	L superior temporal region
Paulesu et al. 1996	NI (5) RD (5)	Letter pairs Korean character pairs	Letter name rhyme matching	Visual similarity (Korean characters)	Active>control	NI>RD	L STG L insula
Rumsey et al. 1997	NI (14) RD (17)	Visual words, pseudowords	Read aloud	Fixation	Active>control	NI>RD	Posterior temporal (including L STG) L fusiform L inferior parietal
						RD>NI	L insula

Table 3–1. Neuroimaging studies comparing adults with reading disorder and nonimpaired adults performing cognitive tasks related to reading or phonological processes *(continued)*

Authors	Subjects (*n*)	Stimuli	Active task	Control	Type of effect	Group effect	Region
						Key findings	
PET (continued)							
Horwitz et al. 1998[b]	NI (14) RD (17)	Words, pseudowords	Read aloud	Fixation	Correlation with angular gyrus activity and other regions	NI>RD	L STG Fusiform/ lingual Inferior frontal areas
Brunswick et al. 1999	NI (6) RD[c](6)	Words, pseudowords	Read aloud[d]	Rest, eyes closed	Active>control	NI>RD	Fusiform/ lingual gyrus (BA 37) Cerebellum
						RD>NI	Premotor areas

Developmental Psychobiology of Reading Disability 75

Table 3–1. Neuroimaging studies comparing adults with reading disorder and nonimpaired adults performing cognitive tasks related to reading or phonological processes (continued)

Authors	Subjects (n)	Stimuli	Active task	Control	Key findings		
					Type of effect	Group effect	Region
PET (continued)							
Brunswick et al. 1999 (continued)	NI (6) RD[c](6)	Words, pseudowords, false fonts	Feature detection[e]	Rest, eyes closed	Active>control	NI>RD	Basal temporal region (including fusiform gyrus) L inferior parietal L inferior temporal L midtemporal
Paulesu et al. 2001[f]	NI (36) RD (36)	Words, pseudowords	Read aloud[d] (18 RD, 18 NI) Feature judgment[e] (18 RD, 18 NI)	Baseline rest False fonts	Conjunction analysis of explicit and implicit task contrasts showing group effects	NI>RD[f]	L STG L midtemporal L fusiform L midoccipital

Table 3–1. Neuroimaging studies comparing adults with reading disorder and nonimpaired adults performing cognitive tasks related to reading or phonological processes *(continued)*

Authors	Subjects (*n*)	Stimuli	Active task	Control	Type of effect	Group effect	Region
						Key findings	
			MEG				
Salmelin et al. 1996	NI (8) RD (6)	Words, nonwords	Silent reading with infrequent probe trial	Prestimulus baseline	Stimulus locked response: 180 ms	NI>RD	L posterior source (near BA 37)
					Stimulus locked response: 200–400 ms	NI>RD	L temporal lobes (near STG)

Table 3–1. Neuroimaging studies comparing adults with reading disorder and nonimpaired adults performing cognitive tasks related to reading or phonological processes (*continued*)

Authors	Subjects (*n*)	Stimuli	Active task	Control	Type of effect	Group effect	Region
						Key findings	
		MEG (*continued*)					
Helenius et al. 1999	NI (10) RD (12)	Words, geometric symbol strings presented in different levels of visual noise	Passive viewing with infrequent probe trial	Prestimulus baseline	Stimulus locked response: 100 ms	NI=RD	Sources within early visual regions
					Words> symbols at 180 ms	NI>RD	Sources near basal temporal region (including fusiform gyrus)
Helenius et al. 2002	NI (10) RD (9)	Speech: syllables with short or long gaps between onset and rhyme	Passive listening Active discrimination of rare deviant syllables[g]	Prestimulus baseline	Amplitude of response within 100 ms to deviant syllable (both tasks)	RD>NI	L STG

Table 3–1. Neuroimaging studies comparing adults with reading disorder and nonimpaired adults performing cognitive tasks related to reading or phonological processes (*continued*)

Authors	Subjects (*n*)	Stimuli	Active task	Control	Key findings		
					Type of effect	Group effect	Region
			MEG (*continued*)				
Helenius et al. 2002 (*continued*)		Nonspeech: rapid pairs of simple tones, complex sounds	Passive listening Active discrimination of rare deviant syllables[g]	Prestimulus baseline	Stimulus locked responses	NI=RD	L/R STG

Table 3–1. Neuroimaging studies comparing adults with reading disorder and nonimpaired adults performing cognitive tasks related to reading or phonological processes (*continued*)

Authors	Subjects (*n*)	Stimuli	Active task	Control	Type of effect	Group effect	Region
			fMRI				
S.E. Shaywitz et al. 1998[h]	NI (32) RD (29)	Line segments	Orientation match	Each task served as a control for the next in the hierarchy	Increasing activity with increasing task demands in the hierarchy	NI>RD	L STG Angular gyrus Striate cortex (BA 17)
		Letter strings	Letter case matching				
		Pseudowords	Rhyme matching				
		Words	Category matching			RD>NI	IFG

Note. fMRI=functional magnetic resonance imaging; IFG=inferior frontal gyrus; L=left; MEG=magnetoencephalography; NI=nonimpaired; PET=positron-emission tomography; R=right; RD=reading disability; STG=superior temporal gyrus.

[a]49 regions examined; region-of-interest analysis.
[b]Same sample as Rumsey et al. 1997.
[c]Remediated.
[d]Explicit reading.
[e]Implicit reading.
[f]Three language groups (French, English, Italian).
[g]/a/ followed by /ta/ vs. /a/ followed by /a/).
[h]17 regions of interest based on previous studies. Stimulus-Task pairings are shown.

1997), but this pattern does not appear in most studies.

Another consistent pattern across studies appears within the visual system when examining activity patterns in response to the presentation of visual words. Across studies involving visual presentation of words or wordlike stimuli (pseudowords), non-impaired adults show increased activity in the vicinity of left fusiform gyrus (basal temporal region BA 37) in a way that adults with reading disorder do not. This general pattern of group differences in response to visual word forms was present even when task instructions were unrelated to the linguistic properties of the stimuli (Brunswick et al. 1999) and was consistently replicated across nonimpaired and dyslexic readers of English, French, and Italian (Paulesu et al. 2001). In a recent review of evidence for the functional contribution of this region during reading tasks, responses in this region were shown to be sensitive to abstract letter information and to common orthographic patterns and thus may reflect a form of learned perceptual expertise for reading (McCandliss et al. 2003).

MEG studies are an important complement to PET and fMRI studies because they provide information about temporal dynamics of activity over the course of the several hundred milliseconds typically required to recognize a word. Whereas fMRI and PET images provide a detailed map of regions activated by a task, MEG provides the opportunity to investigate the time course of activity within these different brain regions.

Contrasting MEG responses between groups of adults with and without reading disorder has identified several converging insights that are fairly consistent across studies. Early responses to visual words typically occur within 100 ms in posterior occipital areas and are equivalent between reading-impaired and nonimpaired subjects. MEG sources located in or near the fusiform gyrus (basal temporal region) show that the earliest differential response between subjects with and without reading disorder while viewing a word does not appear until 180 ms after stimulus onset (Salmelin et al. 1996). In nonimpaired adult readers, this early MEG response is sensitive to differences between visual words and a set of control symbol stimuli, but this effect is absent in subjects with reading disorder, who show equivalent responses to words and control symbols (Helenius et al. 1999). Approximately 200–400 ms after stimulus onset, a second group difference emerges over left posterior temporal regions (near superior temporal gyrus), in which nonimpaired readers show stronger responses than do subjects with reading disorder while reading words (Salmelin et al. 1996). This same region also shows differences in MEG responses between reading-disordered and nonimpaired subjects listening to speech sounds, suggesting a role in phonological analysis (Helenius et al. 2002).

Another important finding involves an examination of how activation patterns within certain brain regions act in a coherent fashion during tasks that involve reading. Horwitz and colleagues (1998) examined this issue in reading-disordered and nonimpaired subjects by performing correlational analyses on fMRI data to examine the extent to which angular gyrus activity was correlated with activity in reading-related areas, such as the left superior temporal gyrus and the fusiform gyrus. Findings indicated that the strength of such correlations was significantly reduced in subjects with reading disorder relative to nonimpaired readers.

Together, the available adult neuroimaging literature provides strong converging evidence across numerous paradigms and imaging methodologies toward a neurobiological profile for reading disorder. This profile is marked by both a disruption of the early response to visual words in the left fusiform region and a tendency toward hypoactivity of posterior temporal regions as subjects engage in a wide range of phonological tasks, including reading words and analyzing the sounds within spoken words. Some studies show clear evidence that individuals with reading disorder have increased activity in other regions (relative to nonimpaired subjects), potentially reflecting some form of compensatory strategy. However, the size and location of such effects appear to change across paradigms, and such activity may be entirely dependent on task demands unique to each experiment. In addition to identifying functional disruptions within cortical regions, adult functional neuroimaging indicates that efficient communication between phonological regions and visual word form analysis regions might be affected in reading disorder (Horwitz et al. 1998).

Several limitations, however, are inherent in the central paradigm used in adult functional neuroimaging studies that directly compare reading-impaired and nonimpaired groups. Reports of functional differences between reading-impaired and nonimpaired adults open some ambiguities for interpretation. For example, the available evidence does not provide a means of discriminating whether a particular functional disruption *preceded* reading difficulties and is thus more likely to have played a causal role, represents a *late-emerging response* to childhood difficulties in reading and phonological processing, or represents functional reorganization typically associated with years of successful reading but absent in the case of reading disabilities. Studies that examine only the final adult outcome of long-term developmental processes provide little insight into whether a given functional disruption represents a fundamental limit on the level of reading skill one might attain or acts as a developmental bias that might be counteracted across the development of reading skill. Such limitations can be addressed via a developmental approach that involves children in cognitive testing and neuroimaging studies during the years in which reading skills are initially developing.

Neuroimaging Studies of Children With Reading Disability

Recent advances in child-friendly, noninvasive imaging procedures, together with a growing interest in the intersection of human development and cognitive neuroscience, have promoted a great deal of progress in imaging the developmental course of several psychiatric disorders (Casey et al. 2001). Table 3–2 highlights key findings from five recent neuroimaging studies of children with reading disorder that span a range of development much closer to the initial emergence of the major symptoms of reading disorder. We consider in this section how this developmental literature provides new insights into the nature of three central points of convergence from the adult literature: 1) significance of left perisylvian functional disruptions, 2) atypical activation patterns in fusiform gyrus, and 3) other findings of compensatory activity.

Table 3–2. Neuroimaging studies of children with reading disorder

Authors	Subjects (n)	Stimuli	Active task	Control task	Effect	Key findings	
						Group effect	Areas
MEG							
Simos et al. 2000a	NI (10)[a]; age 8–16 RD (11)[b]; age 10–17	Pseudoword pairs[c]	Rhyme match	Prestimulus baseline	Strength of magnetic source solution	NI>RD	L perisylvian
						RD>NI	R perisylvian
						NI=RD	L basal temporal regions (including fusiform gyrus)
Simos et al. 2000b	NI (8)[a]; age 8–16 RD (10)[b]; age 10–17	High-frequency words[d]	Visual word recognition	Prestimulus baseline	Strength of magnetic source solution	RD	Perisylvian sources: R>L
						NI	Perisylvian sources: L>R
						NI=RD	L basal temporal (near fusiform gyrus)

Table 3–2. Neuroimaging studies of children with reading disorder (*continued*)

Authors	Subjects (*n*)	Stimuli	Active task	Control task	Effect	Group effect	Areas
						Key findings	
			fMRI				
Georgiewa et al. 1999[e]	NI (17); age 14 RD (17); age 14 German	Symbol strings Pseudowords Frequent words Frequent words	Passive viewing Silent reading Silent reading Move onset to end, add "ein" (silently)		Pseudowords> symbol strings	NI>RD	L IFG
					Phoneme manipulation task (words)> passive viewing (symbols)	NI>RD	L IFG
Temple et al. 2001	NI (15); age 8–12 RD (24); age 8–12	Line segments Letter pairs	Rhyme match: letters	Visual match: letters	Active>control	NI>RD	L perisylvian (including L STG) L occipitoparietal
						RD>NI	L IFG
			Visual match: letters	Visual match: line segments	Active>control	NI>RD	L mid/superior occipital R precuneous cingulate

Table 3–2. Neuroimaging studies of children with reading disorder *(continued)*

Authors	Subjects (*n*)	Stimuli	Active task	Control task	Effect	Group effect	Areas
			fMRI (continued)			**Key findings**	
B.A. Shaywitz et al. 2002	NI (74)[f]; age 7–17 RD (70)[g]; age 7–18	Visual stimuli unique to each task	Pseudowords: rhyme match Words: category match	Line segments: orientation match	Active (both tasks)> control	NI>RD	LH and RH perisylvian; frontal regions
					Positive correlation of brain activity (active> control) and decoding skill	All subjects combined	L basal temporal (including L fusiform)

Note. fMRI=functional magnetic resonance imaging; IFG=inferior frontal gyrus; L=left; LH=left hemisphere; MEG=magnetoencephalography; NI=nonimpaired; R=right; RD=reading disability; RH=right hemisphere; STG=superior temporal gyrus.
[a]>80th percentile decoding.
[b]<30th percentile decoding.
[c]Visually presented.
[d]From 2nd-grade texts.
[e]Investigators contrasted Stimulus-Task pairings shown.
[f]>39th percentile decoding.
[g]<25th percentile decoding.

Functional Disruptions in
Left Perisylvian Regions

Temple and colleagues (2001) used fMRI to scan a group of 8- to 12-year-old children with and without reading disorder. They contrasted letter rhyming with visual matching of letters or line segments. A previous adult neuroimaging paradigm (Paulesu et al. 1996) showed hypoactivity in left superior temporal gyrus of adults with reading disorder relative to nonimpaired adults. As summarized in Table 3–2, results of this child study provided a critical replication of a central finding from the adult literature—as phonological task demands increased, children with reading disorder showed less recruitment of left perisylvian regions (including left superior temporal gyrus). This finding was present even when controlling for IQ across groups, suggesting that it is somewhat specific to phonological processing.

A similar effect was found in a large cross-sectional developmental study of 70 children with reading disorder and 74 non-impaired children ranging in age from 7 to 17 (B. A. Shaywitz et al. 2002). Cortical responses to two active reading tasks designed to engage phonology and reading skills (pseudoword rhyme match, word category match) compared with a baseline task designed to control for visual stimulation and decision making. Results showed significantly less activity for children with reading disorder in a range of areas, including the superior temporal gyrus. Other regions (see Table 3–2) also showed reduced activity for children with reading disorder relative to nonimpaired readers, raising the question of specificity in the functional disruption of the left perisylvian region during the development of reading.

In contrast, a comparison of children with and without reading disorder in Germany (Georgiewa et al. 1999) showed no evidence to support left perisylvian functional disruption. Instead, evidence from two separate tasks that emphasized phonological processes in reading showed reduced activity in left inferior frontal regions for children with reading disorder relative to nonimpaired children.

Additional results from a series of developmental MEG studies, however, successfully replicated the central finding of left posterior functional disruption. One of these studies examined MEG responses to high-frequency words from second-grade texts (Simos et al. 2000b), and another examined MEG responses to a visual pseudoword in a rhyme judgment task (Simos et al. 2000a). Children with reading disorder consistently showed less activation in left perisylvian regions than did nonimpaired children across both visual reading tasks, generally replicating the adult MEG findings. Furthermore, the children with reading disorder showed an atypical pattern of greater recruitment of right perisylvian regions when reading words; this activation was not present in an additional task involving listening to auditory words (Simos et al. 2000b), suggesting a pattern of compensatory recruitment.

These studies present support for the hypothesis that one of the most consistent effects found in brain imaging studies of dyslexic adults—left perisylvian functional disruptions related to phonological processing—is also present earlier in development, while reading skills are still developing. This finding presents the possibility that functional disruption of left perisylvian regions may play a causal role in the atypical development of reading skills and suggests that such findings are not merely a compensatory response or learning effect emerging as a consequence of reading difficulties.

Basal Temporal Regions

Several of the developmental neuroimaging studies presented in Table 3–2 provide an important contrast with the adult reading disorder literature concerning the left fusiform gyrus within the basal temporal region. As reviewed in the adult MEG studies earlier, individuals with reading disorder and nonimpaired readers show different responses to visual words within 200 ms localized to the left basal temporal region near the fusiform gyrus. This pattern does not emerge, however, in MEG contrasts between children with and without reading disorder. When familiar words are presented, responses in this region are equivalent across these two groups of children, in terms of both signal strength and the latency at which activity in this region reaches its peak (Simos et al. 2000b). A similar pattern of results has been reported for pseudowords presented to children in a rhyming task (Simos et al. 2000a).

This developmental difference in fusiform findings in reading disorder is potentially informative in understanding the differential roles left perisylvian regions and left fusiform (basal temporal) regions play in typical and atypical reading development. In skilled adult readers, responses to visual words are differentiated from other visual stimuli (i.e., geometric symbols) within 200 ms of stimulus onset (Tarkiainen et al. 1999). Such responses likely represent a form of perceptual expertise in which a region of extrastriate cortex has become sensitive to specific qualities of visual words, such as the abstract patterns of information that govern how letters are grouped together into visual word forms. It has been proposed that the perceptual expertise that supports such early responses to visual words and pseudowords develops slowly over the course of several years before reaching skilled adult levels (for review, see McCandliss et al. 2003). Under this developmental framework, the functional responses of the fusiform gyrus region to words are what differentiate adults with and without reading disorder, more likely reflecting learning over the course of years of literacy experience rather than a form of functional abnormality in left fusiform gyrus regions per se.

Table 3–2 also provides results of a brain–behavior correlation analysis in children with and without reading disorder spanning ages 7–18 (B. A. Shaywitz et al. 2002). This analysis indicated a significant relation between reading skill (as measured by decoding ability) and the degree of activity in left fusiform gyrus during word and pseudoword reading tasks. Children with the highest level of reading skill tended to have the most robust activity in the region centered on the left fusiform gyrus. Importantly, this relation held true for both children with reading disorder and nonimpaired children, suggesting that the degree to which this region responds to visual words changes over the course of skill acquisition. Thus, improvements in reading skill may be systematically related to increased activity in this region in response to visual words.

Regions of Increased Activity in Reading Disorder

The patterns of increased cortical recruitment in reading disorder also can be informative for understanding atypical development. The developmental studies summarized in Table 3–2 provide insight into cortical areas that children with reading disorder recruit *more* than do nonimpaired children as well as areas they recruit less. As was seen in a review of adult imaging studies, a review of the child imaging studies showed some evidence of regions of greater activity for children with reading disorder across different activation paradigms. For example, both adults and children with reading disorder showed increases in left inferior frontal regions in a study by Temple et al. (2001), but other studies have shown the opposite effect (Georgiewa et al. 1999).

In MEG studies, children with reading disorder show a robust tendency to recruit right perisylvian regions to a greater extent than either their nonimpaired counterparts or their own recruitment of left perisylvian regions. This pattern was consistent across two independent MEG studies, one that involved reading high-frequency familiar words and another that involved reading pseudowords. In an additional experiment that involved listening to high-frequency words, however, children with and without reading disorder showed equivalent responses in left and right superior temporal gyrus regions, suggesting that the group differences are somewhat specific to reading.

A similar finding of increased activity associated with reading disability emerged from brain–behavior correlation analysis from the B.A. Shaywitz et al. (2002) child study. Negative correlations were evident between reading skill and the magnitude of activity in right occipitotemporal regions. This effect was characterized by the poorest readers showing an increased tendency to recruit right hemisphere regions when reading familiar words and making semantic category judgments (B.A. Shaywitz et al. 2002). A similar negative correlation between reading skill and right fusiform gyrus activity has been replicated in a group of nonimpaired children aged 6–22 years (Turkeltaub et al. 2003).

Across several studies summarized in Table 3–2, children with reading disability showed reliable patterns of atypical recruitment, typically involving right hemisphere homologues of brain regions critical for skilled reading. These consistent patterns of right hemisphere recruitment are not present in the adult literature, suggesting that this pattern of right hemisphere recruitment in subjects with reading disorder may be specific to earlier stages of reading development.

In general, childhood neuroimaging studies of reading impairments provide several key insights into the nature and developmental roles of the central findings from the adult literature. First, it appears that patterns of compensatory activity change rather dramatically over the course of development, such that compensatory patterns in young or reading-disabled children involve right perisylvian regions and/or right occipitotemporal regions (including right fusiform), a pattern that is absent in adults with reading disability, who tend to show increased activity in left frontal regions. Developmental data on patterns of activity in the left basal temporal regions suggest that the adult findings of functional differences between reading-impaired and nonimpaired adults may reflect a gradually developing form of perceptual expertise related to developing reading skills. Such learning is perhaps not unlike expertise in face processing described by Scott and Nelson (see Chapter 2 in this volume). Finally, the developmental data indicate that functional disruptions of left perisylvian regions may act as an early, persistent, and potentially causal factor over the course of development of reading disability. This conclusion, however, is somewhat limited by the fact that most of the children in these developmental studies had already been exposed to several years of formal schooling and reading experience before entering each study.

Infant Studies of Speech Processing and Risk for Reading Disorder

One line of developmental research on reading impairments has begun to examine potential evidence for functional abnormalities early in the development of cortical systems related to phonology via event-related potential (ERP) responses to speech sounds in infants. A longitudinal study conducted in Finland (Guttorm et al. 2001) examined 3- to 5-day-old infants' ERP responses to simple speech sounds. This study used the high heritability rates associated with reading disability (Gayan and Olson 2001) to contrast groups of infants with and without familial risk for reading disorder. Familial risk (parental history of reading disability) for reading disorder consistently yields actual incidence of reading deficits in more than one-third of high-risk children (Gilger et al. 1991; Pennington and Lefley 2001). Group contrasts showed distinct ERP effects for children with a familial risk of reading disability, characterized by greater amplitudes and extended durations of ERP responses over right hemisphere sites for particular speech stimuli (e.g., "ga").

A similar 8-year longitudinal study (Molfese 2000) examined the relation between ERP responses to speech sounds in infancy and reading abilities in these same children 8 years later. This study started with no a priori predictors of differences between infants, but instead used multivariate discriminant function analyses to relate childhood reading scores to amplitude and latency estimates for infant ERP recordings in a post hoc fashion. The analyses were capable of classifying infants, on the basis of their ERP data, into one of three childhood outcome groups (control, poor, or dyslexic) with greater than 75% accuracy. Findings from these studies provide clear evidence that reading impairments are accompanied by some form of subtle functional disruption related to speech processing that is present very early in development.

Anatomical Contributions

Based on the notion that regional cellular properties influence computational specialization in local networks, several research efforts have attempted to link functional disruptions in cortical regions to cellular abnormalities in these regions. Evidence for cellular differences has been reported but is typically based on small sample sizes (i.e., $n < 10$). Nonetheless, several postmortem case studies have found ectopias, dysplasias, and microgyria (Galaburda et al. 1985); glial scarring (Humphreys et al. 1990); and minicolumn abnormality (Casanova et al. 2002) in the perisylvian regions of a set of patients with previously diagnosed dyslexia. However, such findings are not exclusive to these regions because cell size differences between dyslexic individuals and control subjects also have been reported in left primary visual cortex (Jenner et al. 1999), lateral and medial geniculate nucleus (for discussion, see Cestnick and Coltheart 1999 and Stein 2001), and most recently, cerebellar regions (Finch et al. 2002).

Other researchers have selectively examined morphological differences in particular brain structures by quantifying variations in size, shape, and asymmetry of entire brain regions. For example, the planum temporale has been a natural region of interest for investigations of abnormalities in language and reading acquisition because this structure is involved in the early auditory analysis of spoken words. Located in auditory association cortex at the posterior end of the sylvian fissure, the planum temporale is engaged in the analysis of spectrotemporal patterns (Griffiths and Warren 2002). Leftward dominance in planum temporale asymmetry is consistently reported in nonimpaired subjects (Preis et al. 1999; Shapleske et al. 1999; Steinmetz 1996; Teszner et al. 1972), whereas reduced planum temporale asymmetry has been reported in dyslexic individuals across several studies (for review, see Habib 2000; Larsen et al. 1990; Morgan and Hynd 1998). However, persistent discrepancies in this literature have led to a host of recent studies that have provided improvements in sample sizes, quantification of subject characteristics, and methods for quantifying brain regions. These more rigorously controlled studies have yielded no significant differences between groups of reading-impaired and nonimpaired adults (Eckert et al. 2002, 2003; Hugdahl et al. 2003; Leonard et al. 2001). Although such null findings cannot rule out the possibility of brain structure differences in reading disorder, such differences are likely to be expressed as biases that fall within the normal range of the nonimpaired population and are likely present in only a subset of subjects with reading disorder.

An important future direction in this work will examine the possibility that morphological variations in multiple brain regions may each contribute a small, but additive, influence on reading ability. One such study examined whole-brain morphological comparisons and more refined phenotypes of dyslexia

(Leonard et al. 2002). Leonard and colleagues (2002) illustrated that different multivariate anatomical criteria are related to different fundamental deficits at different stages of development.

Another important area of research on potential structural differences between subjects with and without reading disorder involves the examination of white matter tracts connecting various brain regions associated with reading and phonology. Diffusion tensor imaging is sensitive to biological properties of white matter tracts by measuring the degree to which water molecules diffuse along the direction of coherent white matter tracts rather than in random directions (a measure called fractional anisotropy; Wieshmann et al. 1999). Recently, diffusion tensor imaging measurements of white matter tracts in bilateral perisylvian regions have shown sensitivity to group differences between adults with and without a history of childhood reading disorder (Klingberg et al. 2000). In left perisylvian regions, the degree of fractional anisotropy was positively correlated with standardized reading scores across the entire range of skill levels.

As discussed earlier, developmental evidence may play an important role in elucidating the causal relation between reading skill and neurobiological measures. Two preliminary reports of unpublished data have recently replicated this effect in children, suggesting that white matter tract differences precede rather than follow reading impairments (Dougherty et al. 2003; Nagy et al. 2002).

Intervention Studies

Given the social significance of developing reading skills in children, rigorous cognitive studies of reading intervention have been abundant. Many studies provide evidence that support the basic claim that children with mild to severe reading impairments can benefit significantly from intervention techniques that involve explicit training and support in phonological awareness and alphabetic decoding skills (Foorman et al. 1998; Torgesen et al. 2001; Vellutino et al. 1996). Such interventions have been shown to produce dramatic improvements for children with reading impairment over the course of one to two semesters of focused intervention.

Combining reading intervention studies with neuroimaging techniques in children can help to address questions about the inherent limitations or plasticity of observed patterns of activity associated with dyslexia. Furthermore, examining the functional reorganization that takes place over the course of an intervention may provide insight into the nature of how an intervention achieves its effect. Some intervention approaches may have a direct effect on the core deficits and the associated abnormal patterns of functional activity, but others may achieve their effects by recruiting compensatory mechanisms. Furthermore, given that children with reading disorder have a tendency to both underactivate some regions involved in normal reading function and overactivate other regions in relation to typically developing readers, an intervention could act to normalize these regions. Accordingly, successful interventions would presumably increase activity in regions that children with reading impairments fail to properly use, as well as reduce activity in regions that are not typically associated with skilled performance of the task, providing that the activation paradigm selected captures the critical aspects of cognitive improvement. Table 3–3 summarizes the details of three recently published studies that combine phonological interventions directed toward children with reading impairments and neuroimaging measures applied both before and after intervention.

One of the first imaging intervention studies (Simos et al. 2002) used MEG to examine neural changes during the visual pseudoword rhyming task described earlier (see "Functional Disruptions in Left Perisylvian Regions"; Simos et al. 2000a) over a 2-month intervention period. Eight reading-impaired children showed pretest MEG measures that replicated the pattern of group differences found in their previous study—the reading-impaired group had both smaller responses over left superior temporal gyrus regions and larger responses over right superior temporal gyrus regions in relation to an age-matched control group of nonimpaired readers. After a 2-month intervention period involving 80 hours of direct intervention with one of two commercial packages (Phono-Graphics and Lindamood Phoneme Sequencing), each child showed large improvements in

Table 3–3. Studies that combine phonological interventions directed toward children with reading impairments and neuroimaging measures applied both before and after intervention

Authors	Subjects (*n*)	Intervention	Behavioral outcome	Neuroimaging results	
				Pretest	Posttest
Aylward et al. 2003	NI[a] (11) RD[b] (10) age 11	Syllable and phoneme awareness, decoding activities, reading (28 hours) vs. NI control[a]	Moderate improvements in decoding skill[c]	fMRI: same/different phoneme judgment for graphemes within pseudowords vs. identity judgment for two consonant strings NI>RD (stronger in LH) for frontal (inferior, mid, superior), parietal (superior, inferior), temporal regions (inferior, mid, AG), and fusiform gyrus	Posttest group differences diminished, associated with both increases in RD and decreases in NI control[a] for inferior, midfrontal gyrus, and superior parietal areas

Table 3–3. Studies that combine phonological interventions directed toward children with reading impairments and neuroimaging measures applied both before and after intervention *(continued)*

Authors	Subjects (*n*)	Intervention	Behavioral outcome	Neuroimaging results	
				Pretest	Posttest
Simos et al. 2002	NI[a] (8), 1/8 ADD RD[b] (8), 6/8 ADD age 7–17	*Phono-Graphics* (*n*=6) or *Lindamood Phoneme Sequencing* (*n*=2) phonological awareness programs (80 hours)	Large improvements on standardized reading test[c]	MEG: rhyme judgment for pairs of visually presented pseudowords NI>RD in sources near L STG RD>NI in sources near R STG	RD: increases in RD activity in L STG, decrease in R homologue NI: stable pre–post responses

Table 3–3. Studies that combine phonological interventions directed toward children with reading impairments and neuroimaging measures applied both before and after intervention *(continued)*

Authors	Subjects (*n*)	Intervention	Behavioral outcome	Neuroimaging results Pretest	Neuroimaging results Posttest
Templeet al. 2003	NI[a] (12) RD[b] (20) age 8–12	Combined treatment: *Fast ForWord Language*—adaptive auditory training for rapid temporal processing and phonemic awareness (45 hours) *Specialized school for dyslexia*	Moderate improvements in word reading, decoding, and passage comprehension[c]	fMRI: rhyming letters *vs.* matching letters: NI>RD in L perisylvian regions (i.e., as in Temple et al. 2001)	Excluding all areas of NI change, RD showed increases in 14 unique brain regions within LH and RH, including L temporoparietal region and BA 37 (near L fusiform gyrus). Changes in temporoparietal activation correlated with changes in auditory language skills but not reading.

Note. ADD=attention-deficit disorder; AG=angular gyrus; fMRI=functional magnetic resonance imaging; L=left; LH=left hemisphere; MEG=magnetoencephalography; NI=nonimpaired; R=right; RD=reading impaired; RH=right hemisphere; STG=superior temporal gyrus.
[a]Nonimpaired group did not receive any intervention.
[b]Intervention.
[c]No control group.

reading scores. Mean standardized reading scores progressed from the 5th percentile before the intervention to the 50th percentile afterward. Such gains are generally consistent with published response rates to well-structured tutorial intervention programs (Torgesen et al. 2001).

Following intervention, reading-impaired children showed significant changes in MEG responses to pseudowords, including both increases in left superior temporal gyrus activity and a decrease in right superior temporal gyrus activity. The eight non-impaired children who did not participate in the intervention showed stable MEG responses over a similar time span.

In an fMRI study conducted with the letter rhyme task described earlier (see "Functional Disruptions in Left Perisylvian Regions"; Temple et al. 2001), Temple et al. (2003) measured changes in functional activity in a group of reading-impaired children participating in a 6-week intervention program (45 hours total). The intervention phase included a commercial computer-training program (*Fast ForWord Language*) in conjunction with a special school curriculum for children with dyslexia. This combination resulted in significant reading improvements. Pretest fMRI results indicated that reading-impaired children showed reduced temporal-parietal activity and inferior frontal activity relative to control subjects. Changes in posttest fMRI results were widespread for the reading-impaired children, including more than 14 brain regions in addition to regions showing shared changes with the nonimpaired group. These regions included a subset typically involved in phonological processes as well as several regions that are not (i.e., cingulate, hippocampus). The magnitude of activation changes in left temporoparietal regions correlated with improvements in oral language, although no such correlation with reading improvements was found.

A third intervention study (Aylward et al. 2003) also showed evidence of changes in neuroimaging profiles for reading-impaired children following an intervention. The 28-hour intervention involved activities that stress "linguistic awareness, alphabetic principle, fluency, and reading comprehension," which resulted in an improvement in standard scores on a measure of reading novel words. A task assumed to isolate grapheme–

phoneme mapping processes was used to probe the effects of treatment on changes in brain activity. In pretest measures, 14 general brain regions showed less activity in the children with reading disorder relative to nonimpaired children, indicating a lack of specificity in the task that potentially complicates interpretation of changes. The intervention group had no significant change in areas previously associated with phonology and reading, such as left perisylvian regions and left fusiform gyrus regions. Some patterns of changes were reported across other cortical regions, although statistical limitations did not allow clear differentiation of whether such changes reflected significant increases in the reading disorder group or significant decreases in the nonimpaired group. The nonspecific nature of the pretest activation patterns and the ambiguities in the nature of the changes that occurred for both groups underscore the importance of well-developed and validated probe tasks in characterizing intervention-based changes in activity.

Together, the convergent results across these initial intervention and neuroimaging studies stand as a form of proof-of-concept demonstration that functional activation differences between those with reading disorder and nonimpaired readers may in some cases prove to be quite malleable in response to effective therapeutic interventions. Such findings show the degree to which activation patterns, under some circumstances, may change dramatically over the course of relatively short-lived experiences. The Simos et al. (2002) and Temple et al. (2003) studies showed that, with interventions, significant change can be induced within the very same cortical regions that have been consistently implicated in adult and child neuroimaging studies as well as within structural and anatomical studies. These findings suggest that interventions can serve to counteract a dominant psychobiological phenotype of reading disability—the tendency for hypoactivation of left perisylvian regions during phonological processing.

MEG methods provide an additional source of information for assessing the effect of interventions in the form of timing information at the millisecond level. In the Simos et al. (2002) study, signs of functional disruption in left superior temporal gyrus persisted even after remediation, as the peak latency of this effect was more than 230 ms slower than that of the nonimpaired group even after the intervention. It is possible that this effect taps into aspects of functional disruptions that are more difficult to change through short-term intervention, such as the fluency of phonological operations.

These initial studies represent a new research paradigm for investigating the relation between specific interventions and specific changes in cortical activity. In theory, such paradigms could help to elucidate specific causal relations between therapeutic interventions and changes in cortical activation patterns associated with core processing deficits in reading disability.

The specific inferences that can be drawn from these three initial studies are limited by several factors, however. For example, none of the three studies included key controls that would be crucial for establishing a causal link between the intervention activities and the observed changes in cortical activity, such as a reading-impaired control group randomized to an alternative intervention. Other challenges involve the selection of appropriate functional activation paradigms and the specificity of results obtained during pre- and posttest measures. In the case of the Aylward et al. (2003) study, the pretest task failed to specifically isolate cortical regions established as critical for grapheme–phoneme processing or to show clear evidence for changes within phonological and graphemic analysis regions for the intervention group. In contrast, the other two studies used tasks that had been validated previously by contrasts between reading-impaired and nonimpaired children and adults and have been found to isolate regions associated with reading and phonological processing. An additional limitation to interpretation comes in the form of intervention results that are nonspecific. In the Temple et al. study, the fact that numerous regions throughout diverse brain regions showed significant changes presents challenges for understanding the specific relation between improvements in ability and changes in particular brain regions. Identifying changes specifically associated with critical improvements in targeted cognitive skills may require additional development of assessment tasks.

Another complication is illustrated by the nature of the pretest contrast in the Simos et al. study. The complexity of the visual pseudoword rhyming task may have precluded children with severe reading disability from engaging in any attempt at phonological analysis. In fact, pretest mean accuracy was at chance performance (51.1%); thus, the pretest task provided no evidence for the types of mental operations the children were engaging, with the possible exception of the increased recruitment of right superior temporal gyrus regions. If this low performance accuracy reflects a complete disengagement in the phonological aspects of the task, perhaps resulting from an inability to read the pseudowords of the task, then interpretations mandated by the evidence of cortical changes are rather limited.

Overcoming such methodological issues will require a better characterization of the relation between performance and activation in both reading-impaired and nonimpaired children (for discussion, see Schlaggar et al. 2002) and the development of tasks that will allow direct comparison of children with reading disorder and nonimpaired children performing at comparable levels. One methodological advance that already has been extensively used in developmental studies of reading disability involves contrasting children who have reading disorder with a younger control group matched for overall reading ability (Goswami and Bryant 1989). Inclusion of such a control group in developmental imaging studies would provide a basis for characterizing pretest differences in children with reading disorder as developmental delays that are similar to the typical development of reading compared with qualitatively different patterns of development.

Conclusion

In summary, the last decade of research on reading disability has produced a great deal of evidence at the cognitive, neural systems, and cellular levels of analysis. Cognitive research has identified a core phonological processing deficit associated with reading disability in both adults and children, as well as a host of other cognitive difficulties that show substantially weaker relations with reading disability. Neuroimaging research relates adult reading disability to particular functional disruptions within and between cortical regions associated with processing visual and phonological information important to reading. Adults with reading disability produce a wide range of cortical responses that diverge from those of nonimpaired readers, including a tendency to underrecruit left perisylvian regions and overrecruit left frontal regions during phonologically demanding tasks and a tendency to show reduced responses to visual words in left basal temporal regions. Some of these phenomena appear to be linked to differences in cellular populations, including subtle disruptions in perisylvian regions that include white and gray matter irregularities, and also may relate to morphological differences in the shape and size of particular gyri.

Throughout this chapter, we argue that examining the *development* of the differences between individuals with reading disorder and nonimpaired readers meaningfully facilitates the description of causal relations between the reviewed findings—as well as the study of the implications of these findings for the purpose of intervention. Evidence from infant ERP studies indicates that some aspects of reading disability, specifically those associated with early responses to speech sounds, are linked to differences between infants with and without familial risk for reading disorder. Because these differences in brain activity precede any substantial exposure to language, they are presumably the result of neuroanatomical biases attributed to genetic influences.

Neuroimaging evidence from children at the age when reading ability and disability first emerge as stable traits shows several important similarities to and differences from the adult literature that are potentially instructive. First, children with reading disorder show the same general pattern of reduced activity in left perisylvian regions in response to phonological demands, suggesting that such atypical patterns may reflect a somewhat stable characteristic of reading disorder responses spanning from infancy to adulthood. In contrast, response patterns in left fusiform gyrus to visual words are similar across children with and without reading disorder, suggesting that the adult difference may be more associated with developmental changes that occur between late childhood and adulthood. We propose that late-emerging differences between individuals with and without reading disorder reflect differences in perceptual expertise associated with years of successful or unsuccessful reading experience, akin to other forms of extensive experience that have been found to modify fusiform responses to classes of stimuli.

Finally, examination of childhood differences between reading-disordered and nonimpaired brain activity shows patterns of compensatory activity that are not found in adults, including increased recruitment in right perisylvian and right fusiform areas. Although the cognitive implications of such patterns of activity are not currently known, such findings indicate that compensatory patterns of activity associated with reading disorder change dynamically across the development of reading skills.

In closing, we observe that the initial studies of childhood reading disorder examining the effect of intensive intervention on cortical responses have reported considerable degrees of plasticity in such responses, especially within areas shown to be hypoactive in the processing of phonological information in childhood and adulthood reading disorder. Carefully engineered intervention protocols appear to counteract the neurobiological biases shown in developmental studies of reading disorder, producing significant changes in reading achievement as well as changes in patterns of cortical activity. Although a host of methodological limitations in the current literature prevent the establishment of direct causal relations between the prescribed intervention activities and the observed changes in cortical activity, many of these challenges in method have been addressed successfully in other imaging studies and other intervention studies. This research soon may provide a framework for systematically studying the causal relations between intervention techniques designed to stress particular principles, such as increasing children's attention to the relation between graphemes and phonemes within word forms, and changes within cortical activation patterns typically associated with reading disability.

References

American Psychiatric Association: Diagnostic and Statistical Manual of Mental Disorders, 4th Edition, Text Revision. Washington, DC, American Psychiatric Association, 2000

Aylward EH, Richards J, Beringer VW, et al: Instructional treatment associated with changes in brain activation in children with dyslexia. Neurology 61:212–219, 2003

Bradley L, Bryant PE: Categorizing sounds and learning to read—a causal connection. Nature 301:419–421, 1983

Bradley L, Bryant PE: Children's Reading Problems. Oxford, UK, Blackwell, 1985

Brunswick N, McCrory E, Price CJ, et al: Explicit and implicit processing of words and pseudowords by adult developmental dyslexics: a search for Wernicke's Wortschatz? Brain 122:1901–1917, 1999

Casanova MF, Buxhoeveden DP, Cohen M, et al: Minicolumnar pathology in dyslexia. Ann Neurol 52:108–110, 2002

Casey BJ, McCandliss BD, Thomas KM: Applications of magnetic resonance imaging to the study of development, in The Handbook of Developmental Cognitive Neuroscience. Edited by Nelson CA, Luciana M. Cambridge, MA, MIT Press, 2001, pp 137–148

Cestnick L, Coltheart M: The relationship between language-processing and visual-processing deficits in developmental dyslexia. Cognition 71:231–255, 1999

Chiappe P, Stringer R, Siegel LS, et al: Why the timing deficit hypothesis does not explain reading disability in adults. Reading and Writing: An Interdisciplinary Journal 15:73–107, 2002

Denkla MB, Rudel RG: Rapid automatized naming: dyslexia differentiated from other learning abilities. Neuropsychologia 14:471–479, 1976

Dougherty RF, Deutsch GK, Siok W, et al: Reading performance in children is correlated with diffusion tensor imaging measurements. Presented at Program 18.4 Society for Neuroscience, New Orleans, LA, November 2003

Eckert MA, Leonard CM, Molloy EA, et al: The epigenesis of planum temporale asymmetry in twins. Cereb Cortex 12:749–755, 2002

Eckert MA, Leonard CM, Richards TL, et al: Anatomical correlates of dyslexia: frontal and cerebellar findings. Brain 126:482–494, 2003

Fast ForWord Language, Oakland, CA, Scientific Learning

Finch AJ, Nicolson RI, Fawcett AJ: Evidence for a neuroanatomical difference within the olivo-cerebellar pathway of adults with dyslexia. Cortex 38:529–539, 2002

Flowers DL, Wood FB, Naylor CE: Regional cerebral blood flow correlates of language processing in reading disability. Arch Neurol 48:637–643, 1991

Foorman BA, Fletcher JM, Francis DJ, et al: The role of instruction in learning to read: preventing reading failure in at-risk children. J Educ Psychol 90:37–56, 1998

Galaburda AM, Sherman GF, Rosen GD, et al: Developmental dyslexia: four consecutive patients with cortical anomalies. Ann Neurol 18:222–233, 1985

Gayan J, Olson RK: Genetic and environmental influences on orthographic and phonological skills in children with reading disabilities. Dev Neuropsychol 20:487–511, 2001

Georgiewa P, Rzanny R, Hopf JM, et al: fMRI during word processing in dyslexic and normal reading children. Neuroreport 10:3459–3465, 1999

Gilger JW, Pennington BF, DeFries JC: Risk for reading disability as a function of parental history in three family studies. Reading and Writing 3:205–217, 1991

Goswami U, Bryant P: The interpretation of studies using the reading level design. Journal of Reading Behavior 21:413–424, 1989

Griffiths TD, Warren JD: The planum temporale as a computational hub. Trends Neurosci 25:348–353, 2002

Guttorm TK, Leppanen PHT, Richardson U, et al: Event-related potentials and consonant differentiation in newborns with familial risk for dyslexia. J Learn Disabil 34:534–544, 2001

Habib M: The neurological basis of developmental dyslexia: an overview and working hypothesis. Brain 123(pt 12):2373–2399, 2000

Helenius P, Tarkiainen A, Cornelissen P, et al: Dissociation of normal feature analysis and deficient processing of letter-strings in dyslexic adults. Cereb Cortex 9:476–483, 1999

Helenius P, Salmelin R, Richardson U, et al: Abnormal auditory cortical activation in dyslexia 100 msec after speech onset. J Cogn Neurosci 14:603–617, 2002

Horwitz B, Rumsey JM, Donohue BC: Functional connectivity of the angular gyrus in normal reading and dyslexia. Proc Natl Acad Sci U S A 95:8939–8944, 1998

Hugdahl K, Heiervang E, Ersland L, et al: Significant relation between MR measures of planum temporale area and dichotic processing of syllables in dyslexic children. Neuropsychologia 41:666–675, 2003

Humphreys P, Kaufmann WE, Galaburda AM: Developmental dyslexia in women: neuropathological findings in three patients. Ann Neurol 28:727–738, 1990

Jenner AR, Rosen GD, Galaburda AM: Neuronal asymmetries in primary visual cortex of dyslexic and nondyslexic brains. Ann Neurol 46:189–196, 1999

Jorm AF: Specific reading retardation and working memory: a review. Br J Psychol 74:311–342, 1983

Klingberg T, Hedehus M, Temple E, et al: Microstructure of temporoparietal white matter as a basis for reading ability: evidence from diffusion tensor magnetic resonance imaging. Neuron 25:493–500, 2000

Larsen JP, Hoien T, Lundberg I, et al: MRI evaluation of the size and symmetry of the planum temporale in adolescents with developmental dyslexia. Brain Lang 39:289–301, 1990

Leonard CM, Eckert MA, Lombardino LJ, et al: Anatomical risk factors for phonological dyslexia. Cereb Cortex 11:148–157, 2001

Leonard CM, Lombardino LJ, Walsh K, et al: Anatomical risk factors that distinguish dyslexia from SLI predict reading skill in normal children. J Commun Disord 35:501–531, 2002

Lindamood Phoneme Sequencing, San Luis Obispo, CA, Lindamood-Bell

Manis FR, Custodio R, Szeszulski PA: Development of phonological and orthographic skill: a 2-year longitudinal study of dyslexic children. J Exp Child Psychol 56:64–86, 1993

McCandliss BD, Noble KG: The development of reading impairment: a cognitive neuroscience model. Ment Retard Dev Disabil Res Rev 9:196–204, 2003

McCandliss BD, Cohen L, Dehaene S: Trends in Cognitive Neurosciences. The visual word form area: expertise for reading in the fusiform gyrus. Trends in Cognitive Neurosciences 7:293–299, 2003

Molfese DL: Predicting dyslexia at 8 years of age using neonatal brain responses. Brain Lang 72:238–245, 2000

Morgan AE, Hynd GW: Dyslexia, neurolinguistic ability, and anatomical variation of the planum temporale. Neuropsychol Rev 8:79–93, 1998

Nagy Z, Westerberg H, Klingberg T: Development of temporal white matter structure correlates with reading ability—a DTI study. Presented at Society for Neuroscience, Orlando, FL, November 2002

National Reading Panel: Teaching Children to Read: An Evidence-Based Assessment of the Scientific Research Literature on Reading and Its Implications for Reading Instruction. Washington, DC, National Institute of Child Health and Development, 2000

Nicholson RI, Fawcett AJ, Dean P: Dyslexia, development and the cerebellum. Trends Neurosci 24:515–516, 2001

Paulesu E, Frith U, Snowling M, et al: Is developmental dyslexia a disconnection syndrome? Evidence from PET scanning. Brain 119:143–157, 1996

Paulesu E, Demonet J-F, Fazio F, et al: Dyslexia: cultural diversity and biological unity. Science 291:2165–2167, 2001

Pennington BF, Van Orden GC, Smith SD, et al: Phonological processing skills and deficits in adult dyslexia. Child Dev 61:1753–1778, 1990

Pennington BF, Lefley DL: Early reading development in children at family risk for dyslexia. Child Dev 72:816–833, 2001

Phono-Graphics, Orlando, FL, Read America

Preis S, Jancke L, Schmitz-Hillebrecht J, et al: Child age and planum temporale asymmetry. Brain Cogn 40:441–452, 1999

Ramus F: Developmental dyslexia: specific phonological deficit or general sensorimotor dysfunction? Curr Opin Neurobiol 13:212–218, 2003

Ramus F, Rosen S, Dakin SC, et al: Theories of developmental dyslexia: insights from a multiple case study of dyslexic adults. Brain 126:841–865, 2003

Rumsey JM, Andreason P, Zametkin AJ, et al: Failure to activate the left temporoparietal cortex in dyslexia. Arch Neurol 49:527–534, 1992

Rumsey JM, Donohue BC, Brady DR, et al: A magnetic resonance imaging study of planum temporale asymmetry in men with developmental dyslexia. Arch Neurol 54:1481–1489, 1997

Rutter M: Prevalence and types of dyslexia, in Dyslexia: An Appraisal of Current Knowledge. Edited by Benton A, Pearl D. New York, Oxford University Press, 1978

Salmelin R, Service E, Kiesila P, et al: Impaired visual word processing in dyslexia revealed with magnetoencephalography. Ann Neurol 40:157–162, 1996

Schlaggar BL, Brown TT, Lugar HM, et al: Functional neuroanatomical differences between adults and school-age children in the processing of single words. Science 296:1476–1479, 2002

Shapleske J, Rossell SL, Woodruff PW, et al: The planum temporale: a systematic, quantitative review of its structural, functional and clinical significance. Brain Res Brain Res Rev 29:26–49, 1999

Share DL, Jorm AF, Maclean R: Temporal processing and reading disability. Reading and Writing: An Interdisciplinary Journal 15:151–178, 2002

Shaywitz BA, Shaywitz SE, Pugh K, et al: Disruption of posterior brain systems for reading in children with developmental dyslexia. Biol Psychiatry 52:101–110, 2002

Shaywitz SE, Shaywitz BA, Pugh KR, et al: Functional disruption in the organization of the brain for reading in dyslexia. Proc Natl Acad Sci U S A 95:2636–2641, 1998

Simos PG, Breier JI, Fletcher JM, et al: Brain activation profiles in dyslexic children during non-word reading: a magnetic source imaging study. Neurosci Lett 290:61–65, 2000a

Simos PG, Breier JI, Fletcher JM, et al: Cerebral mechanisms involved in word reading in dyslexic children: a magnetic source imaging approach. Cereb Cortex 10:809–816, 2000b

Simos PG, Fletcher JM, Bergman E, et al: Dyslexia-specific brain activation profile becomes normal following successful remedial training. Neurology 58:1203–1213, 2002

Stanovich KE: Matthew effects in reading: some consequences of individual differences in the acquisition of literacy. Reading Research Quarterly 21:360–407, 1986

Stein J: The magnocellular theory of developmental dyslexia. Dyslexia 7:12–36, 2001

Steinmetz H: Structure, functional and cerebral asymmetry: in vivo morphometry of the planum temporale. Neurosci Biobehav Rev 20:587–591, 1996

Tallal P: Auditory temporal perception, phonics, and reading disabilities in children. Brain Lang 9:182–198, 1980

Tarkiainen A, Helenius P, Hansen PC, et al: Dynamics of letter string perception in the human occipitotemporal cortex. Brain 122:2119–2132, 1999

Temple E, Poldrack RA, Salidis J, et al: Disrupted neural responses to phonological and orthographic processing in dyslexic children: an fMRI study. Neuroreport 12:299–307, 2001

Temple E, Deutsch GK, Poldrack RA, et al: Neural deficits in children with dyslexia ameliorated by behavioral remediation: evidence from functional MRI. Proc Natl Acad Sci U S A 100:2860–2865, 2003

Teszner D, Tzavaras A, Gruner J, et al: Right-left asymmetry of the planum temporale; apropos of the anatomical study of 100 brains [in French]. Rev Neurol (Paris) 126:444–449, 1972

Torgesen JK, Rashotte CA, Greenstein J, et al: Academic difficulties of learning disabled children who perform poorly on memory span tasks, in Memory and Learning Disabilities: Advances in Learning and Behavioral Disabilities. Edited by Swanson HL. Greenwich, CT, JAI Press, 1987, pp 305–333

Torgesen JK, Alexander AW, Wagner RK, et al: Intensive remedial instruction for children with severe reading disabilities: immediate and long-term outcomes from two instructional approaches. J Learn Disabil 34:33–58, 2001

Turkeltaub PE, Gareau L, Flowers DL, et al: Development of neural mechanisms for reading. Nat Neurosci 6:767–773, 2003

Vellutino FR, Scanlon D, Sipay ER, et al: Cognitive profiles of difficult-to-remediate and readily remediated poor readers: early intervention as a vehicle for distinguishing between cognitive and experiential deficits as basic causes of specific reading disability. J Educ Psychol 88:601–638, 1996

Wieshmann UC, Clark CA, Symms MR, et al: Reduced anisotropy of water diffusion in structural cerebral abnormalities demonstrated with diffusion tensor imaging. Magn Reson Imaging 17:1269–1274, 1999

Wolf M: Naming, reading, and the dyslexias: a longitudinal overview. Annals of Dyslexia 34:87–115, 1984

Chapter 4

Developmental Psychobiology of Gilles de la Tourette's Syndrome

Kathy A. Gallardo, M.D., Ph.D.
James E. Swain, M.D., Ph.D.
James F. Leckman, M.D.

Tic disorders have been the subject of speculation for at least the past 300 years. Despite the overt nature of tics and decades of scientific scrutiny, our ignorance concerning their causes and determinants remains great. Notions of cause have ranged from "hereditary degeneration" (p. 26) to the "irritation of the motor neural systems by toxic substances, of a self-poisoning bacteriological origin" (p. 39) to "a constitutional inferiority of the subcortical structures...[that] renders the individual defenseless against overwhelming emotional and dynamic forces" (p. 51) (Kushner 1998). In this chapter, we briefly survey the clinical features of Tourette's syndrome and related disorders before considering the available information about the potential role of genetic and environmental factors and the growing body of evidence implicating cortico-striato-thalamo-cortical circuits in the pathobiology of this syndrome.

Symptoms and Natural History

Tourette's syndrome is a neuropsychiatric disorder of development. A subclass of tic disorders, it is characterized by the pres-

This work was supported in part by National Institutes of Health grants MH493515, MH61940, RR06022, and RR00125 and the encouragement of the Tourette Syndrome Association.

ence of sudden stereotyped movements and vocalizations termed *motor* and *phonic tics,* respectively. These motor and phonic tics of Tourette's syndrome may be transient or chronic, and they are notable for their capacity to wax and wane in severity (Robertson et al. 1999). Motor tics often precede vocal tics in onset, and they usually begin between ages 3 and 8 years with transient periods of intense eye blinking or facial grimacing. Phonic tics may begin as early as age 3 years, but they often lag behind the onset of motor tics by several years and are typified by repetitive bouts of sniffing or throat clearing. In uncomplicated cases, motor and phonic tic severity peaks early in the second decade of life, with many patients showing a marked reduction in tic severity by age 19 or 20 (Leckman et al. 1998). However, the most severe cases of Tourette's syndrome persist into adulthood. Extreme forms of this illness involve forceful bouts of self-injurious motor tics, such as hitting or biting and socially stigmatizing coprolalic utterances (e.g., shouting obscenities, racial slurs) and gestures.

Motor and phonic tics occur in bouts over the course of a day and wax and wane in severity over the course of weeks to months (Peterson and Leckman 1998). The bouts are characterized by brief periods of stable intertic intervals of short duration, typically 0.5–1.0 seconds, and interbout intervals may last from minutes to hours over the course of a day. Understanding the processes that govern the timing of tic expression may clarify both neural events occurring in millisecond time scales and the natural history of tic disorders that occurs over the first two decades of life.

Tics are more than intermittent series of involuntary motor discharges. They are frequently associated with antecedent sensory phenomena described as "premonitory" urges, which are experienced as nearly irresistible and, in rare cases, painful. In some individuals with Tourette's syndrome, these urges are a major source of impairment (Kurlan et al. 1989; Leckman et al. 1993). A momentary sense of physical relief or a generalized abatement of inner tension often follows performance of a tic. In addition, evidence indicates that auditory or visual cues may trigger tics, suggesting the potential engagement of these sensory pathways in the induction of tic behaviors (A.J. Cohen and Leckman 1992). Other salient features of tics include the individual's ability to suppress tics for brief periods. Fatigue and stress or any emotional excitement can transiently exacerbate tic expression. However, activities that require focused attention and fine motor control, such as reading aloud, playing a musical instrument, playing certain sports, and, in one well-documented case, performing surgery, commonly are associated with transient improvements in tics. Finally, tics can occur during sleep, but they are much diminished, which distinguishes them from other movement disorders.

Patients with Tourette's syndrome commonly have various comorbid conditions, including obsessive-compulsive disorder (OCD), hyperactivity, attention-deficit/hyperactivity disorder (ADHD), and learning disabilities. When present, these coexisting conditions can add greatly to the morbidity associated with Tourette's syndrome and detract from the patient's overall quality of life (Carter et al. 2000; Peterson et al. 2001a; Spencer et al. 1998).

Epidemiology and Genetics

Reported prevalence rates of Tourette's syndrome vary by age, sex, ethnicity, and method of assessment. At present, the best estimate of the prevalence of Tourette's syndrome is approximately 1% of schoolchildren between ages 5 and 17 years, with many more children experiencing lesser variants (Robertson 2003; Snider et al. 2002).

Genetic studies in twins and families provide compelling evidence that genetic factors are implicated in vertical transmission in families with a vulnerability to Tourette's syndrome and related disorders (Pauls 2003). The pattern of vertical transmission in family members suggests major gene effects, and results of segregation analyses accord with models of autosomal transmission set against a polygenic background. Historically, efforts to identify susceptibility genes within these high-density families with traditional linkage strategies have met with limited success. However, investigators studying a large French-Canadian family have reported evidence for linkage at 11q23 (Merette et al. 2000). Nonparametric approaches with families in which two or more siblings are affected with Tourette's syndrome also have been undertaken. This sib-pair approach is suitable for diseases with an unclear mode of inheritance, and it has been used successfully in studies of other complex disorders, such as type 1 diabetes mellitus and essential hypertension. In one sib-pair study of Tourette's syndrome, two areas were suggestive of linkage, one on chromosome arm 4q and another on chromosome arm 8p ("A Complete Genome Screen in Sib Pairs Affected by Gilles de la Tourette Syndrome: The Tourette Syndrome Association International Consortium for Genetics," 1999).

Identity-by-descent approaches have been used in populations in South Africa and Costa Rica. These techniques assume that a few so-called founder individuals contributed the vulnerability genes that are now distributed within a much larger population. The South African study implicated regions near the centromere of chromosome 2 and on 6p, 8q, 11q, 14q, 20q, and 21q (Simonic et al. 1998). The marker in the French-Canadian family (Merette et al. 2000) that was associated with the highest LOD score was the same marker for which significant linkage disequilibrium with Tourette's syndrome was detected in the South African population.

Several candidate genes have been assessed in people with Tourette's syndrome, including various dopamine receptors (*DRD1, DRD2, DRD4,* and *DRD5*), the dopamine transporter, various noradrenergic genes (*ADRA2A, ADRA2C,* and *DBH*), and a few serotoninergic genes (*5HTT*) (Comings 2001). Genetic variation at any one of these loci is unlikely to be a major source of vulnerability to the disorder, but in concert, these alleles could have an important cumulative effect.

In addition, several cytogenetic abnormalities have been reported in Tourette's syndrome families [3 (3p21.3), 7 (7q35–36), 8 (8q21.4), 9 (9pter), and 18 (18q22.3)]. Among the more recent findings, Verkerk et al. (2003) reported the disruption of the contactin-associated protein 2 gene on chromosome 7. This gene encodes a membrane protein located in a specific compartment at the nodes of Ranvier of axons. The authors hypothesized that disruption or decreased expression of this gene leads to an altered distribution of the potassium channels, thereby influencing neural conduction and/or repolarization of action potentials. However, future research is needed to confirm the accuracy and relevance of this finding.

In summary, the nature of the vulnerability genes that predispose individuals to develop the disorder is unknown. Many genes probably have a role. Clarity about the nature and normal expression of even a few of the susceptibility genes in Tourette's syndrome is likely to provide a major step forward in understanding the pathogenesis of this disorder. Future progress also could depend on identification of characteristic, biologically established, endophenotypes that are closely associated with specific vulnerability genes. Endophenotypes are measurable aspects of human psychiatric disorders that can either be used in linkage analyses as quantitative traits, be modeled in animals with the disease, or both. Promising endophenotypes include neurocognitive, neurophysiological, and neuroanatomical measures and patterns of treatment response.

Environment

Various epigenetic factors have been implicated in the pathogenesis of Tourette's syndrome, including gestational and perinatal insults, sex hormones, autoimmune mechanisms, and psychosocial stressors. For example, perinatal hypoxic and ischemic events appear to increase the risk of developing Tourette's syndrome (Burd et al. 1999; Whitaker et al. 1997) by unknown mechanisms. Male sex is also a risk factor, but the observed gender bias is puzzling. Although this male predominance could be due to genetic mechanisms, frequent male-to-male transmissions within families appear to rule out the presence of an X-linked vulnerability gene. The increased number of males affected has led to the hypothesis that androgenic steroids during critical periods in fetal development may play a role in the later development of Tourette's syndrome (Peterson et al. 1992).

A stress diathesis model of pathogenesis is frequently invoked to explain the emergence or exacerbation of tic disorders because of the strong clinical association with stressful life events. Stress-related neurotransmitters and hormones also have been implicated in Tourette's syndrome. In support of this possibility, data suggest that Tourette's syndrome patients may have a heightened reactivity of the hypothalamic-pituitary-adrenal axis and noradrenergic sympathetic systems as compared with healthy control subjects (Chappell et al. 1996; Findley et al. 2003; Leckman et al. 1995).

Finally, the past decade has seen the reemergence of the hypothesis that postinfectious autoimmune mechanisms contribute to the pathogenesis of some cases of Tourette's syndrome and OCD. Speculation concerning a postinfectious etiology for tic disorder symptoms dates from the late 1800s (Kushner 1998). It is well established that group A β-hemolytic streptococci (GABHS) can trigger immune-mediated disease in genetically predisposed individuals. Rheumatic fever is a delayed sequela of GABHS, occurring about 3 weeks after an inadequately treated upper respiratory tract infection. Inflammatory lesions involving the joints, heart, and/or central nervous system characterize rheumatic fever. The central nervous system manifestations are referred to as Sydenham's chorea. In addition to chorea, some patients with Sydenham's chorea have motor and phonic tics and obsessive-compulsive and ADHD symptoms, suggesting that, at least in some instances, these disorders may share a common etiology.

Swedo and colleagues (1998) proposed that pediatric autoimmune neuropsychiatric disorder associated with streptococcal infection (PANDAS) represents a distinct clinical entity and includes cases of Tourette's syndrome and OCD. In PANDAS, it is postulated that although GABHS is the initial autoimmunity-inciting event, viruses, other bacteria, or noninfectious immunological responses are capable of triggering subsequent symptom exacerbations. Several prospective longitudinal studies are under way to examine the relation between newly acquired GABHS infections and other immune activators. If confirmed, the link between common childhood infections and these lifelong neuropsychiatric disorders is tantalizing and may lead to the development of novel treatments.

Neural Substrates of Habit Formation and Tics

Current concepts have focused attention on the neural substrates of habit formation as being crucial for a deeper understanding of Tourette's syndrome (Leckman 2002). Habits are assembled routines that link sensory cues with motor action. The ability to learn complex behaviors and their subsequent performance becomes easier with repetition. As such, habits are enormously adaptive and part of a common evolutionary heritage that we share with other vertebrates as we engage in goal-directed behavior. The mechanisms of habit acquisition are poorly understood, but extant data suggest the involvement of neural loops that connect the basal ganglia with the cortex and thalamus (Graybiel and Canales 2001; Mink 2001).

Excitatory corticofugal projections to the basal ganglia are glutamatergic and originate largely from layer V pyramidal neurons throughout the neocortex. These projections maintain a degree of topographical organization in their course through the basal ganglia and are thought to provide the basis for functional segregation of information in the form of multiple pathways. Differential characterization may be based on macroscopic targets, as in the direct, indirect, and subthalamic pathways, or may reflect more subtle neuroanatomical and neurochemical organization, as in the striosomal and matrisomal pathways. Figure 4–1 depicts the anatomical features of the cortico-striato-thalamo-cortical circuits, and Tables 4–1 and 4–2 summarize current speculations concerning the molecular and structural origins of tics and related behaviors.

In primates, the basal ganglia comprise several extensively interconnected subcortical nuclei: the striatum (caudate and putamen), globus pallidus, subthalamic nucleus (STN), and substantia nigra (Figure 4–1). The caudate and putamen are the primary input structures, and the pars interna of the globus pallidus and the pars reticulata of the substantia nigra are the primary output structures of the basal ganglia. Intermediate structures within the basal ganglia include the STN, pars externa of the globus pallidus, and pars compacta of the substantia nigra. Motor, sensorimotor, association, and inhibitory neural circuits course through the basal ganglia, forming multiple, partially overlapping but largely "parallel" circuits that direct information from the cerebral cortex to the subcortex and then back again to specific regions of the cortex. Although various anatomically and functionally related cortical regions provide input into a particular circuit, each circuit in turn refocuses its projections back onto

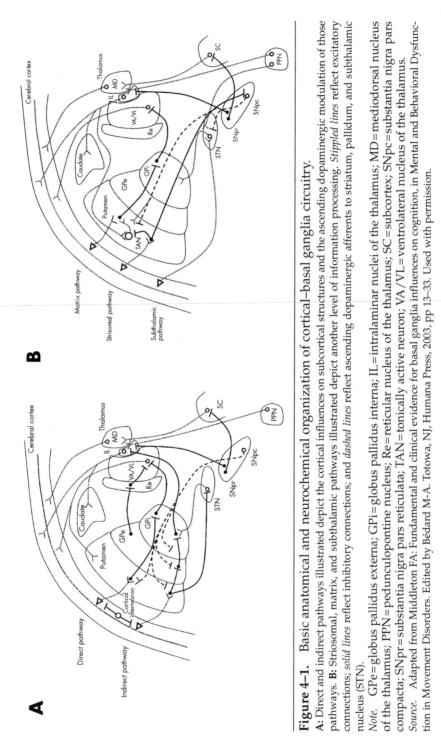

Figure 4–1. Basic anatomical and neurochemical organization of cortical–basal ganglia circuitry.

A: Direct and indirect pathways illustrated depict the cortical influences on subcortical structures and the ascending dopaminergic modulation of those pathways. **B:** Striosomal, matrix, and subthalamic pathways illustrated depict another level of information processing. *Stippled lines* reflect excitatory connections; *solid lines* reflect inhibitory connections; and *dashed lines* reflect ascending dopaminergic afferents to striatum, pallidum, and subthalamic nucleus (STN).

Note. GPe=globus pallidus externa; GPi=globus pallidus interna; IL=intralaminar nuclei of the thalamus; MD=mediodorsal nucleus of the thalamus; PPN=pedunculopontine nucleus; Re=reticular nucleus of the thalamus; SC=subcortex; SNpc=substantia nigra pars compacta; SNpr=substantia nigra pars reticulata; TAN=tonically active neuron; VA/VL=ventrolateral nucleus of the thalamus.

Source. Adapted from Middleton FA: Fundamental and clinical evidence for basal ganglia influences on cognition, in Mental and Behavioral Dysfunction in Movement Disorders. Edited by Bédard M-A. Totowa, NJ, Humana Press, 2003, pp 13–33. Used with permission.

Table 4–1.   Neurobiology of Tourette's syndrome: potential tic
initiators

Tic initiators—Potential mechanisms leading to specific subsets of
medium spiny projection (MSP) neurons becoming active, which
could account for the specific character of individual tics.

Normal physiological events—A cough that persists well after a "cold"
has run its course (A.J. Cohen and Leckman 1992) may involve
abnormalities in sensory motor gating (Swerdlow et al. 2001).

Normal perceptual stimuli—Specific tics being cued by specific
perceptual stimuli in the environment—hearing a specific word and
needing to respond with an orchestrated bout of tics (A.J. Cohen and
Leckman 1992)—may involve abnormalities in sensory motor gating
(Swerdlow et al. 2001).

Immunological stimuli—Antibodies that recognize surface molecules
on MSP neurons and promote signal transduction and abnormal
activation (Kirvan et al. 2003).

a discrete subset of cortical regions initially contributing to that
circuit's input. Within the basal ganglia and thalamus, these mi-
crocircuits appear to be anatomically segregated from others that
course through the same macroscopic structure—hence, the con-
ceptualization of these overlapping pathways as being parallel.
Although the number of anatomically and functionally discrete
pathways remains the subject of controversy, the current consen-
sus holds that cortical–basal ganglia circuitry has at least three
components, those originating from and projecting back to sensorimotor, association, and limbic cortices. Each of these loops
may be further subdivided into multiple specialized modular
units that are distributed according to highly ordered and repetitive patterns. For example, the sensorimotor loop has a somatotopic organization in each of its component nuclei, such that
projections from the sensorimotor and motor cortex relating per-
ceptions and movements of the right arm converge on medium
spiny projection (MSP) neurons in the striatum that specialize in
this same anatomical region. A similar somatotopic organization
is seen in the globus pallidus and thalamus.

There are two major pathways through the basal ganglia,
arising from different cellular populations of the striatum (Figure

Table 4–2. Neurobiology of Tourette's syndrome: potential tic facilitators

Tic facilitators—Mechanisms that could potentially facilitate the emergence of tics and sustain their expression but likely do not account for the specific character of individual tics.

Failure of sensory gating (Swerdlow et al. 2001)—Peripheral or central mechanisms that could enhance the physiological effect of specific sets of sensory events.

Dopaminergic hyperinnervation of the striatum (Singer 1992; Singer et al. 2002)—An overactive dopamine transporter system in the striatum, resulting in a decrease in tonic dopamine levels, could account for exacerbation of tics by stimulant medications. Alternatively, environmental stimuli, such as stress or anxiety, could increase phasic bursts of higher-than-normal levels of dopamine because of the overactive transporter system. In addition to direct effects on medium spiny projection (MSP) neurons, this mechanism also could affect the functioning of the tonically active interneurons of the striatum that may play a role in orchestrating the formation of habits.

Imbalance between striosomes and matrisomes in the striatum (Canales and Graybiel 2000)—Possibly mediated by stress or excitement that leads to activation of regions of the limbic cortex, which, in turn, activates the striosomal pathway, leading to an imbalance. However, the viability of this hypothesis has been challenged (see text section "Neural Substrates of Habit Formation and Tics").

Diminished activity of the subthalamic nucleus (G.M. Anderson et al. 1992a, 1992b)—Levels of glutamate have been diminished in the pars interna of the globus pallidus, which may reflect diminished activity of the subthalamic nucleus, which could lead to a disinhibition of thalamocortical projections.

Disinhibition or hyperexcitability of cortical neurons (Ziemann et al. 1997)—Possibly caused by a loss of cortical interneurons during development (S.A. Anderson et al. 2001) or a genetic defect that increases cortical excitability (Verkerk et al. 2003). Either of these mechanisms might lead to MSP neurons becoming abnormally active.

4–1A): a direct pathway and an indirect pathway. The *direct* pathway facilitates motor, emotive, or cognitive action plans by disinhibiting thalamocortical projections. This disinhibition is the result of glutamatergic cortical neurons activating γ-aminobutyric acid (GABA)ergic MSP neurons in the striatum. This activation leads to the inhibition of GABAergic basal ganglia output neurons in the internal segment of the globus pallidus and substantia nigra pars reticulata. The inhibition of these inhibitory neurons then results in the disinhibition of a select group of thalamocortical projection neurons. The *indirect* pathway involves the external segment of the globus pallidus and the STN. By adding an additional inhibitory segment, the indirect pathway can have the opposite effect of inhibiting the expression action plans.

Imposed on the anatomical topography of the basal ganglia circuitry is a complex neurochemical organization, such that neurotransmitter-specific compartments exist, allowing for multiple integrative and regulatory controls of cerebral cortical input. The various neurotransmitters and neuromodulators in the basal ganglia, particularly in the striatum, appear to facilitate learning and habit formation on the basis of sensorimotor, memory-related, or conditional cues.

Cortical projection neurons to the striatum are also known to segregate into two structurally similar, but neurochemically distinct, compartments termed *striosomes* and the *extrastriosomal matrix* (Figure 4–1B). These compartments differ with respect to their cortical inputs. Whereas cortical afferents to striosomal MSP neurons comprise primarily limbic and prelimbic inputs from anterior cingulate and orbitofrontal cortices, MSP neurons situated in the matrix are the targets of primary motor and sensorimotor cortical neurons (Eblen and Graybiel 1995). Precisely how these two compartments interact is not clear. However, the localization of cholinergic tonically active neurons (TANs) and aspiny GABAergic neurons at the boundary between striosomes and the matrix suggests that they may play a role in modulation of information between the two compartments.

Based largely on work from the Graybiel laboratory, the response of subsets of MSP neurons in the striatum has been found to be frequently dependent on a particular series of perceptual cues and environmental conditions, suggesting that a coordinated striatal response is acquired through learning and experience

(Blazquez et al. 2002). Electrophysiological neuron population recordings, in which the activity of multiple MSP neurons is recorded simultaneously, have begun to clarify the role of the striatum and related brain circuits in the learning and production of habitual or automatic behavioral responses. Recently, Graybiel and colleagues performed chronic recordings from ensembles of electrodes in the sensorimotor areas of rat striatum during cued learning tasks (Jog et al. 1999). Interestingly, large-scale changes in recruitment and firing patterns of these neurons occurred during behavioral acquisition, indicating that neuronal response patterns change with procedural learning and remain stable with continued performance of the task.

The TANs and fast-spiking aspiny interneurons are also implicated in playing a role in habit formation. The TANs appear to be exquisitely sensitive to salient perceptual cues because they signal the networks within the cortico–basal ganglia learning circuits when these cues arise (Blazquez et al. 2002). The TANs are responsive to dopaminergic inputs from the substantia nigra, and these signals likely participate in the computation of the perceived salience (reward value) of the perceptual cues along with excitatory inputs from midline thalamic nuclei (Suzuki et al. 2001). The fast-spiking aspiny interneurons of the striatum are electrically coupled via gap junctions that connect adjacent dendrites. Once activated, these fast-spiking neurons can inhibit many striatal projection neurons synchronously (Koos and Tepper 1999). The characteristic electrophysiological properties of the striatal fast-spiking neurons (e.g., irregular bursting with stable intraburst frequencies) are reminiscent of temporal patterning of tics (Peterson et al. 1998). These fast-spiking interneurons are also very sensitive to cholinergic agents, suggesting that they are functionally related to the TANs (Koos and Tepper 2002).

Once the complex modulation of the excitability of the fast-spiking interneurons and the TANs is better understood in relation to their capacity to influence large numbers of striatal projection neurons in both the matrix and the striosomes, it is likely that a deeper understanding of the factors that govern the selective hypersensitivity of patients with Tourette's syndrome to specific perceptual cues will be at hand. Like habits, tic action sequences often arise from a heightened and selective sensitivity to environmental cues from within the body or from the outside world (Table 4–1). These perceptual cues include the premonitory feelings or urges that are momentarily relieved with the performance of tics or compulsions.

Indirect support for the relevance of the complex modulation of the excitability of the fast-spiking interneurons and the TANs to the study of tics also comes from emerging data concerning the balance between the activities of the medium spiny GABAergic projection neurons in the striosomes and the matrix of the striatum. For example, under normal circumstances, the peak metabolic activity occurs in the matrix compartment (matrix>striosome) (Brown et al. 2002). However, when this balance is reversed (striosome>matrix), animals can show ticlike orofacial stereotypies (Canales and Graybiel 2000). The repetitive behaviors that typify stereotypy range from repetitions of single or multiple movements (motor stereotypies) to repetitive, inflexible patterns of attention and planning that resemble tics and other symptoms seen in Tourette's syndrome and related forms of OCD. In the animal studies, the motor responses examined included sudden head and limb movements, sniffing, grooming and rearing, and oral movements such as licking and nibbling in response to cocaine and other psychostimulants and dopamine agonists.

This model of tics (stereotypies) as being the consequence of an imbalance between striosomal and matrix activity has many attractive features, including the fact that the major cortical inputs to the striosomes arise from stress-sensitive limbic regions, which could account for the increase in tics seen during periods of emotional stress or excitement (Table 4–2). However, recent data raise questions about aspects of this hypothesis. In particular, data from Graybiel's group have shown that the selective destruction of TANs and a marked shift in the striosome–matrix balance did little to alter the number of stereotypies seen in response to psychostimulants and dopamine agonists (Saka et al. 2002).

Alternative models for the neural origins of tics include that proposed by Mink (2001), which similarly invokes the intricate internal organization of basal ganglia circuitry but postulates that the organizing principle for involuntary motor behavior corresponds most closely to dysregulated firing of MSP neurons in the matrix (also known as *matrisomes*) via the direct pathway (Figure 4–1A). These matrisomes receive motor and somatosensory cortical inputs and project to basal ganglia output nuclei (Graybiel et al. 1994). According to Mink, a mechanism invoking repeated selective activation of matrisomes is the most parsimonious explanation for the pattern of stereotyped motor output seen with tics. Experimental evidence in support of this hypothesis comes from Alexander and DeLong (1985), who showed that microstimulation of discrete striatal foci in awake monkeys evoked ticlike stereotyped movements of individual body parts. These foci were presumed striatal output neurons because the effect of microstimulation was abolished after microinjection of ibotenic acid into striatum, producing fiber-sparing lesions.

Some combination of these models will likely provide the best account of the neural substrate of tics. In particular, activation of specific, anatomically distinct subcircuits in the direct pathway that involve matrisomal MSP neurons may be key to the expression of individual simple tics, but the elaboration of complex ensembles of movements and vocalizations may well require the organizational wiring of striatum by TANs and fast-spiking aspiny interneurons. Specifically, growing evidence indicates that the fast-spiking GABAergic aspiny interneurons provide a strong feedforward inhibition of the MSP neurons, whereas the lateral interaction between MSP neurons results in a powerful feedback system (Plenz 2003). These two systems with their independent temporal dynamics and steady-state behaviors are likely to be major determinants of the manner in which cortical inputs are processed.

Other portions of these cortico-striato-thalamo-cortical loops also may be involved in the pathobiology of Tourette's syndrome. Prime candidates include the STN, globus pallidus, substantia nigra, and prefrontal cortex. Lesions to any of these structures can produce unwanted motor output. For example, lesions of the STN produce involuntary movements of contralateral limbs (hemiballism and hemichorea). However, the movement patterns produced typically do not have the same stereotyped character as seen in Tourette's syndrome, and this difference may favor a mechanism that leads to the discrete overactivity of a specific set of striatal matrisomes.

As with habits and stereotypies, ascending dopaminergic pathways may play a key role in the consolidation and performance of tics. Evidence for abnormal dopamine neurotransmission comes from the clinical observations that although blockade of dopamine receptors with neuroleptic drugs suppresses tics in most patients, the use of dopamine-releasing drugs may precipitate or exacerbate tics (Scahill et al. 2000). Indeed, it appears that some Tourette's syndrome patients release more dopamine intrasynaptically in response to amphetamine compared with control subjects without Tourette's syndrome (Singer et al. 2002). In addition, studies of monozygotic twins indicated that developmental shifts in the balance of tonic-phasic dopaminergic tone occurred as a result of epigenetic differences, and the density of dopamine D_2 receptors may influence or be influenced by the severity of Tourette's syndrome (Wolf et al. 1996). In addition, the potential for widespread activation of dopaminergic projections from the substantia nigra following limbic activation of striosomes suggests another possible mechanism of habit formation. Such activation may occur through inhibition of GABAergic interneurons (or pars reticulata cells) terminating on dopaminergic cells and dendrites (Grace and Bunney 1995; Haber et al. 2000). These observations, as well as the key role of dopaminergic inputs on TANs, continue to place ascending dopaminergic pathways in a central role in efforts to understand the neural substrates of tics, habits, and stereotypies (Aosaki et al. 1994).

Neuropathological Studies

The published literature on Tourette's syndrome neuropathology is limited to no more than seven presumed Tourette's syndrome cases. Although these studies generally implicated cortico-striato-thalamo-cortical circuits, the data are far from definitive; two findings deserve comment. First, Singer (1992) reported findings from four cases in which a large increase in [^{3}H]-mazindol binding occurred, which is presumably a reflection of an elevated number of dopamine transporter sites and likely an indicator of increased dopaminergic innervation of the striatum. This finding has been replicated in vivo in two small series of patients in which single photon emission computed tomography (SPECT) and the ligand [^{123}I]2 β-carbomethoxy-3 β-(4-iodophenyl)tropane ([^{123}I]β-CIT) were used (Malison et al. 1995; Muller-Vahl et al. 2000). If there is a dopaminergic hyperinnervation of the striatum, this hyperinnervation could potentially contribute to a general increased vulnerability for subsets of matrisomes to become selectively activated in response to specific stimuli (Table 4–2). However, dopaminergic hyperinnervation of the striatum may not be a universal finding in Tourette's syndrome because one subsequent report failed to replicate this finding despite using the same SPECT ligand and similar procedures (Stamenkovic et al. 2001).

Second, G.M. Anderson et al. (1992a, 1992b) reported a series of neurochemical findings in the same four cases studied by Singer (1992). The most striking finding was a dramatic reduction in the levels of glutamate in the globus pallidus and the substantia nigra pars reticulata that was interpreted as reflecting a loss of input from the STN. Because the STN input to these basal ganglia output structures is excitatory and because increased activity in the GABAergic output neurons leads to inhibition of the thalamocortical projections, a loss of glutamatergic input from the STN would lead to a general tendency for the thalamocortical projections to become disinhibited and thus facilitate ticlike behaviors (Table 4–2).

Single Photon Emission Computed Tomography, Positron-Emission Tomography, and Magnetic Resonance Spectroscopy Studies

Metabolism and blood flow studies generally have implicated disturbances in cortico-striato-thalamo-cortical circuits in the pathophysiology of Tourette's syndrome. The most consistent findings in these positron-emission tomography (PET) and SPECT studies have involved the basal ganglia (Gerard and Peterson 2003). For example, Braun et al. (1995) found decreased glucose use in the ventral striatum. Similarly, most blood flow studies have reported reduced perfusion either of the globus pallidus and putamen or of the basal ganglia as a whole, suggesting that metabolism and blood flow in the basal ganglia are probably reduced in Tourette's syndrome adults relative to healthy control subjects. However, this finding also may be a result of the efforts of the patients to suppress their tics in the scanner, as shown in the Peterson et al. (1998) study. Some of these reports also described regions of cortical activation or deactivation, but little consistency has been found across studies.

Investigators also have examined the functional coupling of various brain regions and found that changes in the coupling of the putamen and ventral striatum with several other brain regions differentiated Tourette's syndrome patients from control subjects. For example, Jeffries et al. (2002) found evidence of functional connections between the motor and lateral orbitofrontal circuits in both Tourette's syndrome patients and control subjects. However, the variance of the connections differed between the two groups. In control subjects, activity in these circuits was negatively correlated (i.e., increased activity in one is associated with relative inactivity in the other), whereas among patients with Tourette's syndrome, activity in the motor and lateral orbitofrontal circuits was positively coupled. These results lend further credence to the hypothesis that altered limbic-motor interactions are a hallmark of this disease.

Radioligand studies of Tourette's syndrome have most commonly focused on characterizing the dopaminergic system in adults with Tourette's syndrome. This focus is based on the efficacy of dopamine antagonists in the treatment of Tourette's syndrome, the ability of dopamine agonists to provoke tic symptoms in some Tourette's syndrome patients, and the unequivocally important role dopamine plays in modulating cortico-striato-thalamo-cortical circuits. Thus far, apart from the possible findings of increased intrasynaptic dopamine release in response to amphetamine (Singer et al. 2002), increased number of transporter sites (Malison et al. 1995; Muller-Vahl et al. 2000), and increased levels of type 2 vesicular monoamine transporters (Albin et al. 2003), studies of the dopaminergic system have produced variable and inconsistent findings. However, this inconsistency may be due to regional differences, with the ventral striatum showing abnormally high levels of dopaminergic innervation.

Other investigators have sought to correlate state-dependent regional activations with tic occurrence. In one study, Stern et al. (2000) found increased activity highly correlated with tic behavior. This activity was detected in a set of neocortical, paralimbic, and subcortical regions, including supplementary motor, premotor, anterior cingulate, dorsolateral-rostral prefrontal, and primary motor cortices; the Broca's area; insula; claustrum; putamen; and caudate. Perhaps it is not surprising that in the one patient with prominent coprolalia, the vocal tics were associated with increased activity in prerolandic and postrolandic language regions, insula, caudate, thalamus, and cerebellum.

Finally, only pilot magnetic resonance spectroscopy (MRS) studies focused on the neuronal marker *N*-acetylaspartate have been completed, again with equivocal results (DeVito et al. 2003).

Experiments of Nature

Tourettism secondary to cerebral malignancies or infarction has been reported in at least nine individuals (Kwak and Jankovic 2002). In most cases, tics developed as a result of injury to the ventral striatum and/or anterior portions of the caudate.

Neurosurgical Interventions

The results of neurosurgical procedures reinforce the functional importance of thalamic regions that are part of these cortical-subcortical loops (Rauch et al. 1995; Vandewalle et al. 1999). A single case study found that high-frequency stimulation of the median and rostral intralaminar thalamic nuclei produced an important reduction in tics. This effect could be the result of the influence of these midline thalamic nuclei on the TANs or on broadly distributed cortical systems and their corticostriatal projections or both. As in other movement disorders, a deeper understanding of the circuitry involved in Tourette's syndrome may lead to specific circuit-based therapies that use deep-brain stimulation to treat refractory cases.

Functional Magnetic Resonance Imaging Studies

Thus far, only one high-resolution study that used functional magnetic resonance imaging of blood oxygenation of brain tissue in a relatively small group of adults with Tourette's syndrome has been published (Peterson et al. 1998). In this study, subjects were asked to alternately suppress their tics or release them voluntarily over 40-second blocks. It was found that tic suppression was associated with activation of regions of prefrontal cortex and caudate nucleus, correlated with deactivations of putamen and globus pallidus. Furthermore, it was found that these signal changes were highly intercorrelated with one another as well as being correlated with tic symptom severity during the week before the scan, as rated by an expert clinician. If confirmed, these findings suggest that prefrontal cortical regions linked to portions of the caudate are crucially involved in tic suppression. Whether these same circuits are involved in normal expression of tics is unknown, although some investigators have sought to alter the activity of the prefrontal areas in an effort to enhance control of tics, with mixed results (George et al. 2001).

Structural Imaging Studies

Although several volumetric magnetic resonance imaging studies have been completed over the past decade, most have involved relatively small numbers (<40) of Tourette's syndrome subjects. Recently, however, Peterson and colleagues (2001b, 2003) and Plessen et al. (in press) have written a series of reports involving more than 150 well-characterized children and adults with Tourette's syndrome. In one report, caudate nucleus volumes were found to be approximately 5% smaller in children and adults with Tourette's syndrome (Peterson et al. 2003). On average, the putamen volumes also were smaller, although this finding did not reach statistical significance. The finding of diminished caudate volumes is consistent with the earlier report of Hyde et al. (1995) that documented smaller caudate volumes in the more severely affected members of monozygotic twin pairs.

Tourette's syndrome subjects also have been reported to have larger cortical volumes in dorsal prefrontal and parieto-occipital regions (Peterson et al. 2001b). In the same study, the orbitofrontal, midtemporal, and parieto-occipital regional cerebral volumes were significantly associated with the severity of tic symptoms. Most recently, this same group of investigators examined the size of the corpus callosum and found that in the context of increasing corpus callosum size from childhood to early adulthood, Tourette's syndrome patients typically have a smaller overall corpus callosum size (Plessen et al., in press). This effect was most marked among children younger than 18 years. Indeed, the corpus callosum in the adults with Tourette's syndrome was larger, on average, than the corpus callosum in control subjects. The size of the corpus callosum also was found to correlate inversely with the severity of motor tics. Taken as a whole, these cross-sectional studies implicate broadly distributed cortical systems as well as basal ganglia structures in the pathobiology of Tourette's syndrome.

Prospective longitudinal studies are needed to examine fully the developmental processes, sexual dimorphisms, and possible effects of medication on these findings. It also will be important to determine whether any of these volumetric findings are predictive of later clinical outcomes. It also should be noted that it is impossible to determine from these data whether observed group differences in regional cortical volumes contributed to the production of tics or whether they were somehow a compensatory response.

Potentially Relevant Neuroimmunological Findings

GABHS-induced acute rheumatic fever is one of the best examples of postinfectious autoimmunity resulting from molecular mimicry between host and pathogen. Sydenham's chorea is the major neurological manifestation of rheumatic fever, but its pathogenesis has remained elusive. Recently, Kirvan et al. (2003) reported that antibodies produced by a 14-year-old girl with rheumatic fever showed specificity for mammalian lysoganglioside and N-acetyl-β-D-glucosamine, an epitope of GABHS carbohydrate. More important, these antibodies also targeted the surface of human neuronal cells and induced calcium/calmodulin-dependent protein kinase II activity. Convalescent sera and sera from individuals with other GABHS disorders in the absence of chorea did not activate this kinase. If confirmed, these findings could provide evidence of how specific matrisomal MSP neurons might be activated in Sydenham's chorea and may lead to a better understanding of other antibody-mediated neuropsychiatric disorders such as Tourette's syndrome (Table 4–1).

Neuropsychological Findings

Although motor and phonic tics constitute the core elements of the diagnostic criteria for Tourette's syndrome, perceptual and cognitive difficulties are also common. These neuropsychological symptoms are potentially informative about the pathobiology of the disorder. Moreover, these associated difficulties can be more problematic for school and social adjustment than the primary motor symptoms.

Neuropsychological studies of Tourette's syndrome have focused on a broad array of functions. Review of the literature suggests that the most consistently observed deficits occur on tasks requiring the accurate copy of geometric designs (i.e., visual-motor integration or visual-graphic ability) (reviewed in Schultz et al. 1998). Even after controlling statistically for visual-perceptual skill, intelligence, and fine motor control, children with Tourette's syndrome continued to perform worse than control subjects on the visual-motor tasks, suggesting that the integration of visual inputs and organized motor output is a specific area of weakness in individuals with Tourette's syndrome. More recent reports have made a case for deficits in executive functions predominantly in the areas of response inhibition and action monitoring, suggesting impairment of the frontal-striatal-thalamic-frontal circuits (Muller et al. 2003).

Neurophysiological Studies

Neurophysiological studies of individuals with Tourette's syndrome have yielded two potentially important findings. The first concerns the use of a startle paradigm to measure inhibitory deficits by monitoring the reduction in startle reflex magnitude when the startling stimulus is preceded 30–500 ms by a weak stimulus, or prepulse. This prepulse inhibition (PPI) of the startle response is an operational measure of sensorimotor gating, which refers to the brain's ability to protect incoming information for very brief periods (Swerdlow et al. 2000). Swerdlow and colleagues (2001) recently confirmed and extended earlier findings indicating that Tourette's syndrome patients have deficits in sensory gating across several sensory modalities. Although PPI abnormalities have been observed across various neuropsychiatric populations, including schizophrenia, OCD, Huntington's disease, nocturnal enuresis, ADHD, Asperger's syndrome, and Tourette's syndrome, perhaps some final common pathways might mediate abnormal movements associated with all of these diseases. Hypotheses to account for abnormal PPI include hypofunctioning GABAergic output of the pallidum or excess dopaminergic input from limbic cortex. These deficits in inhibitory gating are consistent with the diminished ability to appropriately inhibit or gate intrusive sensory, cognitive, and motor information and might lead to the induction of tics in response to normal, but poorly gated, sensory input (Table 4–1).

Second, motor system excitability has been investigated in vivo by means of single- and paired-pulse transcranial magnetic stimulation (TMS). Following a single TMS pulse to the motor cortex and the corresponding muscle contraction, the electromyography is silent for a very brief period, reflecting the general degree of inhibitory control within the sensorimotor loop. However, a paired-pulse TMS measures intracortical excitability and reflects the degree of inhibitory and facilitatory control within the motor cortex following a subthreshold prepulse. Studies to date in groups of patients with Tourette's syndrome have indicated that the cortical silent period is shortened in Tourette's syndrome and that intracortical excitability is frequently seen in children with ADHD with a comorbid tic disorder (Moll et al. 1999; Ziemann et al. 1997).

Future Perspectives

Animal and human studies of habits, tics, and stereotypies have advanced in breadth, sophistication, and scope during the past decade, and the number of groups engaged in this work has grown to a point at which a "critical mass" of investigators is poised to have a significant effect on our understanding of habits, tics, and related behaviors. Despite enormous progress, the complexity of these systems in primates and humans is formidable (Holt et al. 1997). A key set of questions posed by the findings in Tourette's syndrome is how best to understand the elaborate interactions between regions of the frontal cortex and the basal ganglia and how these interactions act in concert to learn and release motor, emotive, and cognitive "action plans." Joint ventures that combine the efforts of investigators at the leading edge of genetics, neuroimmunology, and the neurosciences (molecular, systems, developmental, behavioral) with those of clinical scholars are needed to sustain and accelerate progress in this field.

Most of the evidence points to the involvement of cortico-striato-thalamo-cortical circuits being crucial for the development of habits, tics, and stereotypies. Despite this convergence, the precise mechanisms involved remain in doubt. Why do tics appear when they do? Why do they wax and wane? Why do they reach a worst-ever point in early adolescence, for most, and become even more severe in adulthood for an unlucky few? These developmental issues are probably crucial to a full understanding of this disorder, or set of disorders.

The developing monoaminergic systems continue to be a major point of focus because they have been repeatedly implicated in highly diverse behavioral and cognitive functions, including habit formation, the induction of stereotypies, and the treatment of tics. Specifically, midbrain dopaminergic neurons play a central role in motor control and attentional processes by direct connections to striatum and prefrontal cortex, respectively. Understanding the timing and maturation of this system and the role it plays in the growth, differentiation, and plasticity of the cortico-striato-thalamo-cortical circuits, in general, and ventral striatal regions, in particular, may shed light on critical windows of vulnerability in the development, timing, and persistence of tics.

Neural ontogeny of the GABAergic systems is also an intriguing area of study germane to the understanding of movement disorders and the suspected role of faulty inhibitory circuitry. Many GABAergic interneurons of the cerebral cortex migrate tangentially from the same embryonic regions in the ganglionic eminence that also give rise to the GABAergic MSP neurons of the striatum (S.A. Anderson et al. 1997). An appealing hypothesis is that adverse events arising at a specific point in development account for the striatal imbalance and intracortical deficits in inhibition seen in some patients with Tourette's syndrome. Furthermore, given the paucity of information on basal ganglia development, this hypothesis may prove to be a rich area of study regarding the multiplicity of afferent systems and integration of sensorimotor and limbic information. Recent studies examining the cellular and molecular mechanisms involved in the early specification of the striatum have begun to identify spatial and temporal restriction patterns involved in developmental gene and protein expression (Hamasaki et al. 2003; Jain et al. 2001). By understanding the molecular switches involved in cell fate, proliferation, and migration and the development of local and specific feedback inhibition between MSP neurons, it may be possible to design therapeutic interventions to halt or reverse potentially neurotoxic events.

The application of computational neural networks also may greatly enhance the emerging conceptual framework of tic disorders. Use of dynamic representations of neuroanatomical and neurochemical circuitry may one day lead to a greater understanding of the brain–behavior interface. Such models are already being applied to the study of cortical–basal ganglia circuitry as it relates to both motor and cognitive information processing (Frank et al. 2001). For example, modeling of tonic or phasic dopaminergic activity, perhaps mediated by D_1 and D_2 receptors in the prefrontal cortex, respectively, may be promising. Tonic inputs may stabilize representations by increasing the signal-to-noise ratio of background compared with evoked prefrontal cortex activity, whereas phasic inputs may signal when new inputs should be encoded or when old representations should be updated in response to salient, reward-predicting data (J.D. Cohen et al. 2002). As new data regarding different cortical regions are incorporated, future models may provide testable hypotheses of how differences in or manipulations of genetics, organization, and pharmacology may lead to a disordered or a cured phenotype.

In examining the available information, fundamental caveats must be kept in mind, including the potential for compensatory change (e.g., What are the neurobiological consequences of having tics?) and the potential that the mental state of the individual at the time of the study could affect the outcome (e.g., What are the effects on the regional activation of the brain if the individual needs to actively suppress his or her tics during the course of an imaging study?). In the future, we can anticipate the deployment of advanced technologies (MRS, diffusion tensor imaging, near-infrared optical spectroscopy, and as-yet-unknown techniques) and the combination of behavioral (habit reversal or tic suppression) and neurophysiological (single- or paired-pulse TMS or PPI of startle) stimuli within the confines of brain imaging devices. These maneuvers will likely yield valuable data to craft meaningful endophenotypes for future genetic studies. Longitudinal studies are needed to address questions of risk and resilience, and ideally these would involve subjects at high genetic risk who have yet to show the characteristic symptoms of Tourette's syndrome. Likewise, the development of valid animal or neurocomputational models would be a major step forward.

References

A complete genome screen in sib pairs affected by Gilles de la Tourette syndrome: The Tourette Syndrome Association International Consortium for Genetics. Am J Hum Genet 65:1428–1436, 1999

Albin RL, Koeppe RA, Bohnen NI, et al: Increased ventral striatal monoaminergic innervation in Tourette syndrome. Neurology 61:310–315, 2003

Alexander GE, DeLong MR: Microstimulation of the primate neostriatum, I: physiological properties of striatal microexcitable zones. J Neurophysiol 53:1401–1416, 1985

Anderson GM, Pollak ES, Chatterjee D, et al: Brain monoamines and amino acids in Gilles de la Tourette's syndrome: a preliminary study of subcortical regions. Arch Gen Psychiatry 49:584–586, 1992a

Anderson GM, Pollak ES, Chatterjee D, et al: Postmortem analysis of subcortical monoamines and amino acids in Tourette syndrome. Adv Neurol 58:123–133, 1992b

Anderson SA, Eisenstat DD, Shi L, et al: Interneuron migration from basal forebrain to neocortex: dependence on dlx genes. Science 278:474–476, 1997

Anderson SA, Marin O, Horn C, et al: Distinct cortical migrations from the medial and lateral ganglionic eminences. Development 128:353–363, 2001

Aosaki T, Graybiel AM, Kimura M: Effect of the nigrostriatal dopamine system on acquired neural responses in the striatum of behaving monkeys. Science 265:412–415, 1994

Blazquez PM, Fujii N, Kojima J, et al: A network representation of response probability in the striatum. Neuron 33:973–982, 2002

Braun AR, Randolph C, Stoetter B, et al: The functional neuroanatomy of Tourette's syndrome: an FDG-pet study, II: relationships between regional cerebral metabolism and associated behavioral and cognitive features of the illness. Neuropsychopharmacology 13:151–168, 1995

Brown LL, Feldman SM, Smith DM, et al: Differential metabolic activity in the striosome and matrix compartments of the rat striatum during natural behaviors. J Neurosci 22:305–314, 2002

Burd L, Severud R, Klug MG, et al: Prenatal and perinatal risk factors for Tourette disorder. J Perinat Med 27:295–302, 1999

Canales JJ, Graybiel AM: A measure of striatal function predicts motor stereotypy. Nat Neurosci 3:377–383, 2000

Carter AS, O'Donnell DA, Schultz RT, et al: Social and emotional adjustment in children affected with Gilles de la Tourette's syndrome: associations with ADHD and family functioning: attention deficit hyperactivity disorder. J Child Psychol Psychiatry 41:215–223, 2000

Chappell P, Leckman J, Goodman W, et al: Elevated cerebrospinal fluid corticotropin-releasing factor in Tourette's syndrome: comparison to obsessive compulsive disorder and normal controls. Biol Psychiatry 39:776–783, 1996

Cohen AJ, Leckman JF: Sensory phenomena associated with Gilles de la Tourette's syndrome. J Clin Psychiatry 53:319–323, 1992

Cohen JD, Braver TS, Brown JW: Computational perspectives on dopamine function in prefrontal cortex. Curr Opin Neurobiol 12:223–229, 2002

Comings DE: Clinical and molecular genetics of ADHD and Tourette syndrome: two related polygenic disorders. Ann N Y Acad Sci 931:50–83, 2001

DeVito TJ, Nicolson R, Williamson PC, et al: Proton MRSI of Tourette syndrome at 3.0 tesla: abnormalities of the cortico-striato-thalamo-cortical circuit, in Proceedings of the International Society for Magnetic Resonance in Medicine, Vol 11, 11th Scientific Meeting, July 2003. Berkeley, CA, International Society for Magnetic Resonance in Medicine, 2003, p 334

Eblen F, Graybiel AM: Highly restricted origin of prefrontal cortical inputs to striosomes in the macaque monkey. J Neurosci 15:5999–6013, 1995

Findley DB, Leckman JF, Katsovich L, et al: Development of the Yale Children's Global Stress Index (YCGSI) and its application in children and adolescents with Tourette's syndrome and obsessive-compulsive disorder. J Am Acad Child Adolesc Psychiatry 42:450–457, 2003

Frank MJ, Loughry B, O'Reilly RC: Interactions between frontal cortex and basal ganglia in working memory: a computational model. Cogn Affect Behav Neurosci 1:137–160, 2001

George MS, Sallee FR, Nahas Z, et al: Transcranial magnetic stimulation (TMS) as a research tool in Tourette syndrome and related disorders. Adv Neurol 85:225–235, 2001

Gerard E, Peterson BS: Developmental processes and brain imaging studies in Tourette syndrome. J Psychosom Res 55:13–22, 2003

Grace AA, Bunney BS: Electrophysiological properties of midbrain dopamine neurons, in Psychopharmacology: The Fourth Generation of Progress. Edited by Bloom FE, Kupfer DJ. New York, Raven, 1995, pp 163–177

Graybiel AM, Canales JJ: The neurobiology of repetitive behaviors: clues to the neurobiology of Tourette syndrome. Adv Neurol 85:123–131, 2001

Graybiel AM, Aosaki T, Flaherty AW, et al: The basal ganglia and adaptive motor control. Science 265:1826–1831, 1994

Haber SN, Fudge JL, McFarland NR: Striatonigrostriatal pathways in primates form an ascending spiral from the shell to the dorsolateral striatum. J Neurosci 20:2369–2382, 2000

Hamasaki T, Goto S, Nishikawa S, et al: Neuronal cell migration for the developmental formation of the mammalian striatum. Brain Res Brain Res Rev 41:1–12, 2003

Holt DJ, Graybiel AM, Saper CB: Neurochemical architecture of the human striatum. J Comp Neurol 384:1–25, 1997

Hyde TM, Stacey ME, Coppola R, et al: Cerebral morphometric abnormalities in Tourette's syndrome: a quantitative MRI study of monozygotic twins. Neurology 45:1176–1182, 1995

Jain M, Armstrong RJ, Barker RA, et al: Cellular and molecular aspects of striatal development. Brain Res Bull 55:533–540, 2001

Jeffries KJ, Schooler C, Schoenbach C, et al: The functional neuroanatomy of Tourette's syndrome: an FDG pet study, III: functional coupling of regional cerebral metabolic rates. Neuropsychopharmacology 27:92–104, 2002

Jog MS, Kubota Y, Connolly CI, et al: Building neural representations of habits. Science 286:1745–1749, 1999

Kirvan CA, Swedo SE, Heuser JS, et al: Mimicry and autoantibody-mediated neuronal cell signaling in Sydenham chorea. Nat Med 9:914–920, 2003

Koos T, Tepper JM: Inhibitory control of neostriatal projection neurons by GABAergic interneurons. Nat Neurosci 2:467–472, 1999

Koos T, Tepper JM: Dual cholinergic control of fast-spiking interneurons in the neostriatum. J Neurosci 22:529–535, 2002

Kurlan R, Lichter D, Hewitt D: Sensory tics in Tourette's syndrome. Neurology 39:731–734, 1989

Kushner HI: Freud and the diagnosis of Gilles de la Tourette's illness. Hist Psychiatry 9:1–25, 1998

Kwak CH, Jankovic J: Tourettism and dystonia after subcortical stroke. Mov Disord 17:821–825, 2002

Leckman JF: Tourette's syndrome. Lancet 360:1577–1586, 2002

Leckman JF, Walker DE, Cohen DJ: Premonitory urges in Tourette's syndrome. Am J Psychiatry 150:98–102, 1993

Leckman JF, Goodman WK, Anderson GM, et al: Cerebrospinal fluid biogenic amines in obsessive compulsive disorder, Tourette's syndrome, and healthy controls. Neuropsychopharmacology 12:73–86, 1995

Leckman JF, Zhang H, Vitale A, et al: Course of tic severity in Tourette syndrome: the first two decades. Pediatrics 102:14–19, 1998

Malison RT, McDougle CJ, van Dyck CH, et al: [123I]Beta-CIT SPECT imaging of striatal dopamine transporter binding in Tourette's disorder. Am J Psychiatry 152:1359–1361, 1995

Merette C, Brassard A, Potvin A, et al: Significant linkage for Tourette syndrome in a large French Canadian family. Am J Hum Genet 67:1008–1013, 2000

Middleton FA: Fundamental and clinical evidence for basal ganglia influences on cognition, in Mental and Behavioral Dysfunction in Movement Disorders. Edited by Bédard M-A. Totowa, NJ, Humana Press, 2003, pp 13–33

Mink JW: Basal ganglia dysfunction in Tourette's syndrome: a new hypothesis. Pediatr Neurol 25:190–198, 2001

Moll GH, Wischer S, Heinrich H, et al: Deficient motor control in children with tic disorder: evidence from transcranial magnetic stimulation. Neurosci Lett 272:37–40, 1999

Muller SV, Johannes S, Wieringa B, et al: Disturbed monitoring and response inhibition in patients with Gilles de la Tourette syndrome and comorbid obsessive compulsive disorder. Behav Neurol 14:29–37, 2003

Muller-Vahl KR, Berding G, Brucke T, et al: Dopamine transporter binding in Gilles de la Tourette syndrome. J Neurol 247:514–520, 2000

Pauls DL: An update on the genetics of Gilles de la Tourette syndrome. J Psychosom Res 55:7–12, 2003

Peterson BS, Leckman JF: The temporal dynamics of tics in Gilles de la Tourette syndrome. Biol Psychiatry 44:1337–1348, 1998

Peterson BS, Leckman JF, Scahill L, et al: Steroid hormones and CNS sexual dimorphisms modulate symptom expression in Tourette's syndrome. Psychoneuroendocrinology 17:553–563, 1992

Peterson BS, Skudlarski P, Anderson AW, et al: A functional magnetic resonance imaging study of tic suppression in Tourette syndrome. Arch Gen Psychiatry 55:326–333, 1998

Peterson BS, Pine DS, Cohen P, et al: Prospective, longitudinal study of tic, obsessive-compulsive, and attention-deficit/hyperactivity disorders in an epidemiological sample. J Am Acad Child Adolesc Psychiatry 40:685–695, 2001a

Peterson BS, Staib L, Scahill L, et al: Regional brain and ventricular volumes in Tourette syndrome. Arch Gen Psychiatry 58:427–440, 2001b

Peterson BS, Thomas P, Kane MJ, et al: Basal ganglia volumes in patients with Gilles de la Tourette syndrome. Arch Gen Psychiatry 60:415–424, 2003

Plenz D: When inhibition goes incognito: feedback interaction between spiny projection neurons in striatal function. Trends Neurosci 26:436–443, 2003

Plessen KJ von, Wentzel-Larsen T, Hugdahl K, et al: Altered interhemispheric connectivity in individuals with Tourette Syndrome. Am J Psychiatry (in press)

Rauch SL, Baer L, Cosgrove GR, et al: Neurosurgical treatment of Tourette's syndrome: a critical review. Compr Psychiatry 36:141–156, 1995

Robertson MM: Diagnosing Tourette syndrome: is it a common disorder? J Psychosom Res 55:3–6, 2003

Robertson MM, Banerjee S, Kurlan R, et al: The Tourette syndrome diagnostic confidence index: development and clinical associations. Neurology 53:2108–2112, 1999

Saka E, Iadarola M, Fitzgerald DJ, et al: Local circuit neurons in the striatum regulate neural and behavioral responses to dopaminergic stimulation. Proc Natl Acad Sci U S A 99:9004–9009, 2002

Scahill L, Chappell PB, King RA, et al: Pharmacologic treatment of tic disorders. Child Adolesc Psychiatr Clin N Am 9:99–117, 2000

Schultz RT, Carter AS, Gladstone M, et al: Visual-motor integration functioning in children with Tourette syndrome. Neuropsychology 12:134–145, 1998

Simonic I, Gericke GS, Ott J, et al: Identification of genetic markers associated with Gilles de la Tourette syndrome in an Afrikaner population. Am J Hum Genet 63:839–846, 1998

Singer HS: Neurochemical analysis of postmortem cortical and striatal brain tissue in patients with Tourette syndrome. Adv Neurol 58:135–144, 1992

Singer HS, Szymanski S, Giuliano J, et al: Elevated intrasynaptic dopamine release in Tourette's syndrome measured by pet. Am J Psychiatry 159:1329–1336, 2002

Snider LA, Seligman LD, Ketchen BR, et al: Tics and problem behaviors in schoolchildren: prevalence, characterization, and associations. Pediatrics 110:331–336, 2002

Spencer T, Biederman J, Harding M, et al: Disentangling the overlap between Tourette's disorder and ADHD. J Child Psychol Psychiatry 39:1037–1044, 1998

Stamenkovic M, Schindler SD, Asenbaum S, et al: No change in striatal dopamine re-uptake site density in psychotropic drug naive and in currently treated Tourette's disorder patients: a [(123)I]-beta-CIT SPECT-study. Eur Neuropsychopharmacol 11:69–74, 2001

Stern E, Silbersweig DA, Chee KY, et al: A functional neuroanatomy of tics in Tourette syndrome. Arch Gen Psychiatry 57:741–748, 2000

Suzuki T, Miura M, Nishimura K, et al: Dopamine-dependent synaptic plasticity in the striatal cholinergic interneurons. J Neurosci 21:6492–6501, 2001

Swedo SE, Leonard HL, Garvey M, et al: Pediatric autoimmune neuro-psychiatric disorders associated with streptococcal infections: clinical description of the first 50 cases. Am J Psychiatry 155:264–271, 1998

Swerdlow NR, Braff DL, Geyer MA: Animal models of deficient sensorimotor gating: what we know, what we think we know, and what we hope to know soon. Behav Pharmacol 11:185–204, 2000

Swerdlow NR, Karban B, Ploum Y, et al: Tactile prepuff inhibition of startle in children with Tourette's syndrome: in search of an "fMRI-friendly" startle paradigm. Biol Psychiatry 50:578–585, 2001

Vandewalle V, van der Linden C, Groenewegen HJ, et al: Stereotactic treatment of Gilles de la Tourette syndrome by high frequency stimulation of thalamus. Lancet 353:724, 1999

Verkerk AJ, Mathews CA, Joosse M, et al: Cntnap2 is disrupted in a family with Gilles de la Tourette syndrome and obsessive compulsive disorder. Genomics 82:1–9, 2003

Whitaker AH, Van Rossem R, Feldman JF, et al: Psychiatric outcomes in low-birth-weight children at age 6 years: relation to neonatal cranial ultrasound abnormalities. Arch Gen Psychiatry 54:847–856, 1997

Wolf SS, Jones DW, Knable MB, et al: Tourette syndrome: prediction of phenotypic variation in monozygotic twins by caudate nucleus D2 receptor binding. Science 273:1225–1227, 1996

Ziemann U, Paulus W, Rothenberger A: Decreased motor inhibition in Tourette's disorder: evidence from transcranial magnetic stimulation. Am J Psychiatry 154:1277–1284, 1997

Chapter 5

Schizophrenia and Neurodevelopment

Susan L. Erickson, Ph.D.
David A. Lewis, M.D.

Schizophrenia is a severe brain disorder that usually produces a lifetime of disability and emotional distress for affected individuals (Lewis and Lieberman 2000). The diagnostic clinical features of the disorder typically appear in the late teens or early 20s, with the average age at onset generally about 5 years earlier in males than in females. Although schizophrenia afflicts approximately 1% of the population throughout the world, the specific factors that give rise to the illness remain elusive.

The risk of developing schizophrenia is directly associated with the degree of biological relatedness to an affected individual (Gottesman 1991); that is, first-degree relatives of an affected individual have a higher risk for the illness than do second-degree relatives, and a monozygotic twin of an individual with schizophrenia is at greater risk than is a dizygotic twin. In addition, when the biological children of individuals with schizophrenia are adopted away, their risk of developing schizophrenia is elevated, as expected for first-degree relatives, and is much higher than the general population rates of schizophrenia present in their adoptive families (Ingraham and Kety 2000; Kety et al. 1971). Furthermore, the offspring of identical twins discordant for schizophrenia have elevated rates of the disorder, independent of whether the parent was affected or unaffected (Gottesman and Bertelsen 1989).

However, because the degree of concordance for schizophrenia among monozygotic twins approaches only 50% (Gottesman

1991), it is clear that genetic liability alone is not sufficient for the clinical manifestation of the illness. Thus, considerations of the etiology of schizophrenia also have included the role of environmental factors. The importance of these factors is shown by the fact that in twin studies, the nonshared environment accounts for almost all of the liability for schizophrenia attributable to nongenetic effects (Tsuang et al. 2001). Many of the environmental events that have been associated with an increased risk for schizophrenia occur during the prenatal or perinatal periods of life. For example, advanced paternal age at the time of conception, maternal influenza during the second trimester of pregnancy, labor and delivery complications, and increased population density at the place of birth and rearing all have been associated with an increased risk for developing schizophrenia later in life (Lewis and Levitt 2002). In addition, individuals who develop schizophrenia are more likely to have had motor abnormalities in early childhood, to have had lower IQ and academic performance in grade school, and to have experienced social difficulties in their early teens than are unaffected siblings or schoolmate control groups (Lewis and Levitt 2002). Thus, the pathogenesis of schizophrenia is considered to represent the confluence of genetic susceptibility and environmental risk factors that alter the biological mechanisms involved in neurodevelopmental processes that transpire prior to the onset of clinical symptoms.

However, given the protean manifestations of schizophrenia, understanding the specific roles that normal and abnormal neurodevelopmental processes play in the illness requires a focus on those aspects of schizophrenia that are central to its pathogenesis. Although psychosis is frequently the most striking clinical feature of schizophrenia, disturbances in critical cognitive processes are now regarded as a core feature of the illness for the following reasons (Elvevåg and Goldberg 2000). First, cognitive abnormalities have been observed in individuals with schizophrenia many years before the onset of the clinical features required for diagnosis (Cosway et al. 2000; Green 1998) as well as in their unaffected siblings (Egan et al. 2001). Second, cognitive abnormalities represent the most disabling and persistent features of the illness (Green 1998). Third, the degree of cognitive impairment may be the best predictor of long-term outcome in individuals with schizophrenia (Green 1996; Harvey et al. 1998).

A variety of cognitive abnormalities have been described in schizophrenia, including disturbances in selective attention (Carter et al. 1992; Cornblatt et al. 1989; Mirsky 1969; Neuchterlein and Dawson 1984) and working memory (Carter et al. 1996; Gold et al. 1997; Keefe et al. 1995; Park and Holzman 1992). Although other explanations are possible, many of these cognitive deficits appear to reflect a disturbance in executive control, the process that facilitates complex information processing and behavior (Posner and Di Girolamo 1998; Shallice 1988) and that includes context representation and maintenance, functions dependent on the dorsolateral prefrontal cortex (DLPFC) (Botvinick et al. 2001; Carter et al. 1999; Cohen et al. 2002). Other domains of investigation also indicate that cognitive abnormalities in schizophrenia are associated with abnormal function of the DLPFC (Goldman-Rakic 1999; Weinberger et al. 2001). For example, under appropriate conditions of cognitive activation, decreased blood flow or glucose utilization in the DLPFC (hypofrontality) appears to be a consistent finding in schizophrenia (Taylor 1996; Weinberger et al. 1986, 1988), although these disturbances are less reliably found in the resting state (Andreasen et al. 1992; Buchsbaum 1990; Gur and Gur 1995). Most interpretations of these results converge on the idea that DLPFC dysfunction in schizophrenia is task specific and related to working memory impairment (Carter et al. 1998; Goldman-Rakic 1987). DLPFC activity is associated with the engagement of executive control during working memory performance (Smith and Jonides 1999), and this is implemented by representing and maintaining the information set required for optimal task performance.

Studies that examined neural activity with functional magnetic resonance imaging (fMRI) (Callicott et al. 1998) indicated that during working memory tasks, subjects with schizophrenia showed an altered relation between DLPFC activation and task difficulty. Under low levels of working memory load, subjects with schizophrenia show activation of the DLPFC, but this activity does not increase in relation to level of load as it does in nonschizophrenic control subjects (Callicott et al. 1999). Under certain conditions in which subjects with schizophrenia and control subjects performed at or close to the same levels, activation of the DLPFC may have been increased in the subjects with schizophrenia (Callicott et al. 2000; Manoach et al. 1999), suggesting that even when subjects with schizophrenia are able to meet the information-processing demands of the task, they do so with reduced efficiency (Weinberger et al. 2001). The central importance of these alterations in DLPFC function to the pathogenesis of the schizophrenia syndrome is supported by the absence of such disturbances in disorders such as major depression (Barch et al. 2003).

Thus, characterizing the development of the neural circuitry of the DLPFC that appears to underlie the maturation of working memory function may be central to understanding the pathogenesis of the schizophrenia syndrome. Because the DLPFC is markedly expanded and differentiated in the primate brain and undergoes a protracted period of postnatal development compared with rodents (Lewis 1997), in this chapter, we focus on studies in macaque monkeys. Specifically, we review the normal postnatal developmental changes that occur in the neural circuitry of the primate DLPFC and consider how these events may inform our understanding of the disturbances of this circuitry in schizophrenia.

Neural Circuitry of the Dorsolateral Prefrontal Cortex

The architecture of the primate DLPFC (Figure 5–1) incorporates the same basic laminar and columnar organization and cell populations common to other neocortical areas, although many fine details show characteristic regional specialization (Lewis et al. 2002). Neuron populations include a) spiny pyramidal cells (shown in blue in Figure 5–1), which release the excitatory neurotransmitter glutamate; and b) nonspiny interneurons (shown in pink in Figure 5–1), which release the inhibitory transmitter γ-aminobutyric acid (GABA). Each of these cell populations can be further subdivided based on their projection patterns and synaptic targets of their axons, the specific gene products that they express, and their morphological features. Many of these subpopulations of DLPFC neurons have been shown to undergo an-

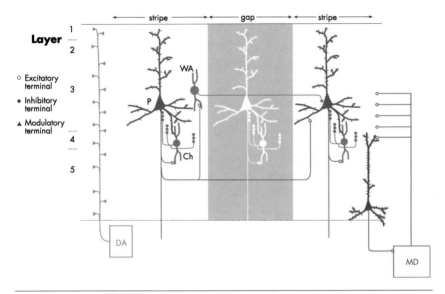

Figure 5–1.   Elements of dorsolateral prefrontal cortex (DLPFC) circuitry implicated in the pathophysiology of schizophrenia.

Cortical layers are indicated by *arabic numerals* at the left of the figure, and the laminar boundaries are indicated by *dashed lines*. Pyramidal neurons (P) of deep layer 3 are shown in *blue*. Two types of inhibitory neurons, the wide arbor (WA) and chandelier (Ch) cells, are shown in *pink*. All three of these cell types form distinctive patterns of connections with respect to the columnar units of information processing ("stripes") in the DLPFC. The pyramidal neurons form connections both within their home column, or stripe, and with remote columns but form relatively few connections with the immediately adjacent regions ("gaps") (Kritzer and Goldman-Rakic 1995; Levitt et al. 1993; Pucak et al. 1996). The pyramidal cells in deep layer 3 are also a significant source of inputs to the small pyramidal cells of layer 6 (shown in *green*) (White 1989), which provide a gateway for descending output from the DLPFC to subcortical targets such as the thalamus (Erickson and Lewis, in press; Giguere and Goldman-Rakic 1988; McFarland and Haber 2002). The WA cells have axonal dimensions that are consistent with forming connections with remote stripes, while skipping the adjacent "gap" regions. In contrast, the Ch neurons form connections exclusively within their home column (Lund and Lewis 1993). Sources of ascending inputs to the DLPFC include dopaminergic (DA) afferents, shown in *yellow,* and afferents from the mediodorsal nucleus of the thalamus (MD), shown in *orange.*

atomical and physiological alterations indicative of changes in their connectivity or activity patterns during a protracted period of postnatal development in primates.

The lengthy period of dynamic modification of the primate DLPFC provides a window of opportunity for any anomaly in the circuitry, even a subtle one, to have its effects amplified as it affects the cascade of developmental events that follow. Thus, when we examine the components of DLPFC circuitry in schizophrenia, which can be done only in postmortem human tissue, for evidence of altered developmental trajectories, we cannot necessarily deduce whether an observed alteration in the disease state is a primary defect or the brain's adaptive response to a defect. However, studies of the normal maturation of different elements of DLPFC circuitry can provide valuable data about the sequence of developmental events and suggest testable hypotheses about their relations. These, in turn, can be used to interpret the postmortem findings. Thus, in the following sections, we review selected aspects of the postnatal development of DLPFC pyramidal neurons and interneurons, and of afferent projections to the DLPFC, in macaque monkeys and consider how each of these findings informs postmortem studies of the analogous neural circuitry components in schizophrenia.

Postnatal Development of Dorsolateral Prefrontal Cortex Pyramidal Neurons

Subclasses of pyramidal neurons can be distinguished by their projection patterns, which may include both local and remote cortical areas, as well as subcortical sites (DeFelipe and Farinas 1992). One population of particular interest is the large pyramids found in deep layer 3 of the DLPFC. These cells form a pattern of local connections that has a distinctive clustered appearance, densely innervating some cortical columns and skipping others (Levitt et al. 1993).

This clustered pattern of intrinsic connections, found in all cortical regions, has been suggested to link columns of neurons sharing some feature of the information processed in those columns (Gilbert and Wiesel 1989). For example, in the primary visual cortex, intrinsic horizontal connections connect columns of cells that show enhanced levels of activity in response to similar stimulus orientation. In the case of the prefrontal regions, it has been suggested that cortical columns linked by horizontal connections share common "memory fields," or locations in the environment essential for spatial working memory (Goldman-Rakic 1995; Lewis and Anderson 1995). In addition to these patchy, local connections, pyramidal neurons of deep layer 3 form connections with more

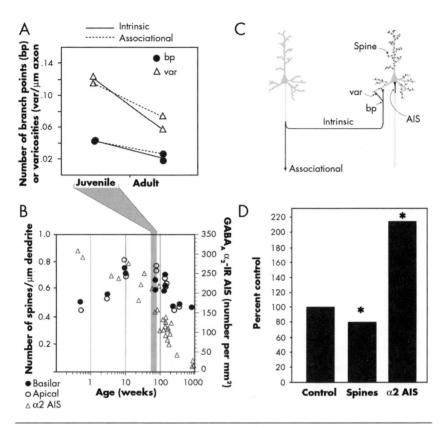

Figure 5–2. Markers of excitatory and inhibitory inputs to pyramidal cells **(C)** change during postnatal development **(A, B)** and are altered in schizophrenia **(D).**

Panel A shows two indices of the complexity of the axon arbors of deep layer 3 pyramidal neurons in juvenile (age 14–21 months) and adult monkeys (adapted from Woo et al. 1997). Both the number of branch points (bp) and the number of varicosities (var), or putative sites of synaptic contacts, are higher in the younger animals compared with adults. Similar observations were made for both intrinsic *(points joined by solid lines)* and associational *(dashed lines)* connections. **Panel B** shows the postnatal development of the density of spines *(circles)*, a measure of the excitatory inputs to pyramidal neurons, and the number of axon initial segments (AIS) immunoreactive for the γ-aminobutyric acid $(GABA)_A$ receptor α_2 subunit *(triangles)*, one index of the inhibitory inputs (adapted from Anderson et al. 1995; Cruz et al. 2003). Spine density measurements were similar on both the apical *(open circles)* and the basilar dendrites *(filled circles)*. The age range *highlighted in gray* in Panel B indicates the specimens that are similar in age to the juvenile animals examined for intracortical axon complexity, shown in Panel A. **Panel D** shows that both spine density and pyramidal neuron (AIS) immunoreactive for the $GABA_A$ α_2 subunit are significantly altered (indicated by *asterisks*) in postmortem material from individuals with schizophrenia compared with control subjects (adapted from Glantz and Lewis 2000; Volk et al. 2002).

distant regions of the prefrontal cortex (Pucak et al. 1996); these are referred to as *associational connections* (Figure 5–2).

Several parameters of both the intrinsic and the associational connections in the monkey DLPFC undergo substantial refinements during postnatal development (Woo et al. 1997). For example, axon complexity appears to decrease significantly during adolescence. Specifically, the branching density of both intrinsic and associational corticocortical axons is lower in adults compared with prepubertal animals (Figure 5–2A). Second, the density of axonal varicosities, or putative sites of synaptic transmission, is lower in adults compared with juveniles for both intrinsic and associational axons (Figure 5–2A). This finding is consistent with ultrastructural studies of the density of all excitatory synapses, which show a plateau at a high density from approximately 3 to 18 months of age and then a marked decrease over the next 18 months until stable adult levels are achieved (Bourgeois et al. 1994). Finally, the tangential dimensions of intrinsic axon clusters diminish between prepubertal and adult ages. These findings show that the axons contributing to local, excitatory circuitry of the DLPFC undergo substantial pruning during adolescence and that the extent of developmental refinements in these intrinsic connections may be greater than for associational connections.

Excitatory synapses onto other excitatory neurons are formed almost exclusively at dendritic spines (DeFelipe and Farinas 1992). Measures of spine density on deep layer 3 pyramidal cells in monkey DLPFC have found that this, too, changes substantially during postnatal development (Anderson et al. 1995). Specifically, spine density is relatively low during early postnatal development, increases to reach its peak by age 3 months, remains elevated to around age 15 months, and then declines over the following 2 years of life (Figure 5–2B). These findings, together with the data on the horizontal connections, provide evidence that excitatory connections emanating from, and terminating on, layer 3 pyramidal neurons in the DLPFC undergo substantial pruning before reaching adult levels.

In addition to developmental alterations in the number of excitatory inputs they receive, pyramidal neurons actively modify their responses to inhibitory input by changing the number or composition of their GABA receptors. For example, in rodents, embryonic $GABA_A$ receptors principally contain α_2 and α_5 subunits, whereas in the adult brain, the α_1 subunit predominates (Fritschy et al. 1994). Studies of $GABA_A$ receptor expression can provide valuable information about the mechanisms available to the pyramidal cell for processing its inhibitory input but do not necessarily provide clues as to the identity of the GABA neuron providing that input. One unique exception, however, is in the case of GABA receptors localized to the axon initial segment (AIS) of pyramidal neurons.

The AIS, the locus of spike generation in neurons, provides a key node for inhibitory control over pyramidal cell output (Cobb et al. 1995). In the adult cortex, most $GABA_A$ receptors containing the α_2 subunit are found in pyramidal cell AIS (Loup et al. 1998). GABA receptors, including the postnatally expressed α_2 subunit, have a higher affinity for GABA, faster activation times, and slower deactivation times than receptors containing the more commonly expressed α_1 subunit (Lavoie et al. 1997). Together, these features have been suggested to confer greater synaptic efficacy for GABA transmission occurring at synapses, including the α_2 subunit.

The prevalence of $GABA_A$ α_2 subunits at the AIS has been shown to undergo substantial modification during postnatal development (Cruz et al. 2003). Figure 5–2B shows the density of pyramidal cell AIS immunoreactive for the α_2 subunit in the DLPFC of monkeys at various ages. The density of α_2-immunoreactive AIS starts out relatively high in the infant animals and then follows a steady decline through adulthood. This decline in the number of α_2-immunoreactive AIS may be interpreted as a decrease in the speed and efficacy of GABAergic transmission at the AIS during postnatal maturation rather than a reduction in the number of GABAergic synapses onto the AIS because the total number of inhibitory synapses and the specialized type of inhibitory synapses at the AIS appear to remain constant over this same period (Bourgeois et al. 1994; Lund and Lewis 1993).

Two interesting observations can be made by direct comparison of α_2-immunoreactive AIS, as a measure of inhibitory input efficacy, and the density of dendritic spines, as a measure of excitatory input, on pyramidal cells during postnatal development. First, during early postnatal development, α_2-immunoreactive AIS has already begun the long decline in density, whereas spine density is increasing. The confluence of these two factors would be consistent with an increase in pyramidal cell activity or output. Second, during later postnatal development, both are decreasing together, perhaps maintaining a plateau of activity as unnecessary excitatory connections are pruned away.

Postmortem studies of the DLPFC in schizophrenia suggest that the developmental trajectories of both excitatory inputs to layer 3 pyramidal cells (as reflected by the density of dendritic spines) and inhibitory activity at pyramidal neuron AIS may be altered in the disease state. As shown in Figure 5–2D, in subjects with schizophrenia, basilar dendritic spine density on deep layer 3 pyramidal cells is reduced by about 20% compared with matched nonschizophrenic control subjects (Garey et al. 1998; Glantz and Lewis 2000), whereas the density of GABA α_2-immunoreactive AIS in schizophrenia is more than double the control value (Volk et al. 2002). These findings suggest a marked disruption in the normal balance between the number of excitatory inputs and the efficacy of inhibition at the AIS in layer 3 pyramidal cells in schizophrenia.

Interestingly, the relative ratio of these markers of excitatory and inhibitory inputs is reminiscent of that present during early postnatal development (see left side of Figure 5–2B). Although it seems unlikely that the findings in schizophrenia represent an arrest of development at such an early stage, these disturbances in schizophrenia may reflect an alteration of DLPFC circuitry that makes it unable to support higher levels of working memory load, rendering the impaired performance in schizophrenia analogous to the immature levels of working memory function seen in children and young monkeys (Diamond, in press). However, despite the apparent importance of GABA inputs to the AIS in regulating the synchronization of pyramidal cell function (Cobb et al. 1995; Klausberger et al. 2003), it must be kept in mind that inhibitory synapses at the AIS account for only about 1% of all GABA synapses on pyramidal cells. Furthermore, as discussed in the following section, the changes in GABA α_2 receptors may be secondary to abnormalities in chandelier cells, as opposed to more primary changes in pyramidal neurons.

Postnatal Development of Dorsolateral Prefrontal Cortex Interneurons

Inhibitory interneurons, like pyramidal cells, can be divided into several subpopulations based on the projection pattern of their axon terminals. Unlike pyramidal cells, however, many of the interneuron types assume a characteristic morphological and biochemical phenotype that allows them to be distinguished with conventional histological preparations rather than invasive tract tracing procedures, facilitating translation between experimental preparations and human postmortem material. Two populations of interneurons that have been linked to positive findings in postmortem studies of individuals with schizophrenia—the wide arbor and chandelier neurons—also have been shown to have changes in the expression of certain biochemical markers during a protracted period of postnatal development.

Wide arbor neurons, abundant in layers 3 and 5, are so named for their broad-reaching axon terminal arbors, which can extend for up to 1 mm from the cell body (Lund and Lewis 1993) (Figure 5–1). Although wide arbor neurons form terminal boutons within the local vicinity of the cell body, or within the parent cell's home column, they appear to be specialized for providing inhibition to cells in other columns of the same cortical module, as defined by the patchy pattern of excitatory connections discussed earlier (Lewis and Gonzalez-Burgos 2000) (Figure 5–3C). Thus, the wide arbor neurons have been described as the prefrontal analogue of the basket cells of visual cortex (Jones and Hendry 1984).

Wide arbor neurons contain the calcium-binding protein parvalbumin, and their terminals can be visualized immunocytochemically with antibodies directed at parvalbumin (Condé et al. 1994). The density of these parvalbumin-immunoreactive terminals changes markedly during postnatal development (Erickson and Lewis 2002), increasing steadily in an almost linear fashion from newborn to adult (Figure 5–3A). The total number of inhibitory synapses, and the axonal arbors of wide arbor cells specifically, appear to remain relatively constant over this same period (Bourgeois et al. 1994; Lund and Lewis 1993), suggesting that developmental changes in the number of parvalbumin-immunoreactive terminals reflect a change in the detectability of wide arbor cell terminals with immunocytochemical techniques, most likely attributable to a change in the amount of parvalbumin protein within the terminals. The function of calcium-binding proteins is believed to be protection of the cell from toxic levels of calcium influx during sustained periods of high activity, and modulation of the amount of such a protein has been suggested to be an index of cellular activity (Celio 1984). Thus, the observed developmental increase in the number of parvalbumin-immunoreactive terminals is consistent with an increase in the activity of wide arbor cells. This implies that inhibitory modulation from one cortical column to another column, which are connected by the patchy intrinsic excitatory projections of layer 3 pyramidal neurons, is maximized near the time of puberty, whereas the number of excitatory connections between these same columns is diminishing.

One interpretation of this combination of developmental events is that communication between cortical columns of the same module simply produces less overall drive in the adult DLPFC compared with the immature state. However, work in the visual system suggests that recruitment of disynaptic inhibition modulates neuronal response properties in a much more complex manner and is a critical component in the shaping of receptive field properties (Hirsch and Gilbert 1991; Tucker and Katz 2003). The data summarized previously indicate that in the DLPFC, developmental alterations in inhibitory modulation of neuronal response properties likely contribute to the late-emerging functional maturity of the region (Alexander and Goldman 1978; Kuroda et al. 1993).

The *chandelier* cell class of inhibitory neuron also shows changes in the expression of biochemical markers during a protracted period of postnatal development. Like the wide arbor neurons, the somata and terminals of chandelier neurons can be visualized with antibodies directed against parvalbumin and a GABA plasma membrane transporter subunit (GAT1) (DeFelipe et al. 1989; Lewis and Lund 1990; Woo et al. 1998). However, the

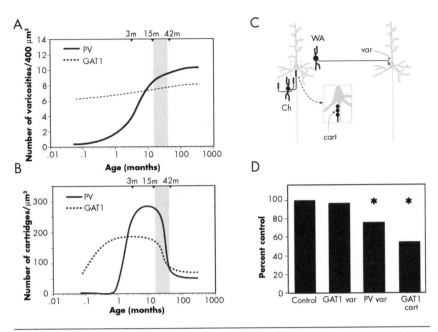

Figure 5–3. Subsets of γ-aminobutyric acid (GABA)ergic terminals **(C)** that are dynamically modified during postnatal development **(A, B)** are also altered in schizophrenia **(D).**

Panel A shows that the density of axon terminals, or varicosities (var), immunoreactive for parvalbumin (PV, *solid line*) increases significantly until puberty in monkeys (age range highlighted in *gray*) (adapted from Erickson and Lewis 2002). Another marker of inhibitory terminals, the GABA plasma membrane transporter (GAT1, *dashed line*), also appears to increase during the same period, but these changes were not significant. These developmental changes are likely to be associated with the wide arbor (WA) class of interneuron **(Panel C). Panel B** shows the postnatal development of cartridges (cart) of the chandelier neuron (Ch; Panel C), visualized with PV*(solid line)* or GAT1 *(dashed line)* (adapted from Cruz et al. 2003). **Panel D** shows that the density of PV-immunoreactive varicosities and GAT1-immunoreactive cartridges are significantly lower (indicated by *asterisks*) in subjects with schizophrenia compared with control subjects (adapted from Lewis et al. 2001; Pierri et al. 1999). In contrast, the density of varicosities labeled with GAT1 in schizophrenic patients was similar to that of control subjects (adapted from Woo et al. 1998).

parvalbumin- and GAT1-immunoreactive terminals of chandelier neurons are readily discriminated from those of wide arbor cells by their distinctive morphology. Chandelier axons form rows of terminal boutons, termed *cartridges,* along the AIS of pyramidal cells (Peters 1984). As noted earlier, synaptic contact at this point of action potential generation provides the chandelier cells with a unique opportunity to regulate pyramidal cell firing

(Cobb et al. 1995; Klausberger et al. 2003). A typical chandelier cell may form cartridges with approximately 250 pyramidal cells over a range of 150–250 μm from the chandelier neuron's cell body (Peters 1984). Work in the hippocampus has shown that a single chandelier neuron can synchronize the firing of multiple pyramidal cells (Cobb et al. 1995). Should this prove to be the case in the cortex, the dimensions of the cortical chandelier cells suggest that they serve to coordinate the activity of excitatory cells within a single column.

During postnatal development, the density of cartridges immunoreactive for either parvalbumin or GAT1 changes markedly in monkeys (Cruz et al. 2003). Although the precise time course differs for the two markers, both indicate low numbers of cartridges in the newborn, an increase to reach a peak before the onset of puberty, and then a decline to adult levels (Figure 5–3B). Because cartridges are readily visualized with the Golgi technique over this period (Lund and Lewis 1993), the changes in parvalbumin- and GAT1-immunoreactive cartridges likely reflect developmental shifts in the amount of each of these proteins, as was suggested for the wide arbor terminals. Interestingly, the peak and subsequent decline in the density of labeled cartridges occur prior to the peak density of labeled wide arbor terminals but appear concomitant with the pruning of intracortical excitatory connections (compare Figure 5–3B with Figure 5–2A and 5–2B). Although other explanations for this temporal coincidence may be possible, we hypothesize that the synchronous firing of a group of pyramidal cells, facilitated by the chandelier neurons, is instrumental in promoting the maintenance of a subset of excitatory connections, whereas others are pruned away.

These developmental changes in wide arbor and chandelier neurons also may be disrupted in schizophrenia, as shown in Figure 5–3D. In postmortem brain specimens from individuals with schizophrenia, the density of GAT1-immunoreactive chandelier neuron axon cartridges in the middle cortical layers is reduced by 50% (Pierri et al. 1999), and the density of parvalbumin-immunoreactive varicosities in these same layers is reduced by about 25% (Lewis et al. 2001). Consistent with these findings, the messenger RNAs (mRNAs) for GAT1 and for glutamic acid decarboxylase, a synthesizing enzyme for GABA, are not detectable in the subpopulation of GABA neurons that express parvalbumin, and the expression level of parvalbumin mRNA in these neurons is below that of control subjects (Hashimoto et al. 2003; Volk et al. 2000, 2001). Together, these findings are consistent with the idea that GABA synthesis and reuptake are reduced in the parvalbumin-containing subpopulation of GABA neurons, which includes chandelier and wide arbor cells, that provide proximal inhibitory input to the AIS and cell soma, respectively, of pyramidal neurons. The specificity of these changes is supported by the observations that the overall density of GAT1-positive varicosities, a marker of all GABA terminals, including the large majority that target the dendrites of pyramidal cells, is unchanged in schizophrenia (Woo et al. 1998) (Figure 5–3D). Consistent with these findings, neither the mRNA levels nor the density of labeled varicosities for calretinin, a calcium-binding protein found in about 50% of cortical GABA neurons that do not contain parvalbumin, appears to be changed in schizophrenia (Hashimoto et al. 2003; Woo et al. 1998). Interestingly, calretinin expression is evident early in prenatal cortical development in primates, whereas parvalbumin expression is not detectable until the postnatal period, observations consistent with the general idea that vulnerability of neural elements in schizophrenia may be related to their developmental trajectory.

Postnatal Development of Ascending Afferents to the Dorsolateral Prefrontal Cortex

In the preceding section, we presented evidence that the density of axon terminals immunoreactive for parvalbumin increases steadily throughout the postnatal development of the DLPFC, until reaching adult levels around the time of puberty. In addition, we interpreted these observations to be consistent with alterations in the activity levels of the wide arbor class of cortical interneurons. An alternative interpretation of this observation is that these changes reflect, at least in part, an ingrowth of afferents from the mediodorsal nucleus of the thalamus (MD), the principal source of ascending projections to the DLPFC and a critical element in the circuitry that subserves working memory (Goldman-Rakic 1987). A proportion of the cells in the MD are immunoreactive for parvalbumin (Jones and Hendry 1989), and parvalbumin appears to be a distinguishing marker for thalamocortical relay cells in certain thalamic nuclei (DeFelipe and Jones 1991). In addition, a variable proportion of parvalbumin-immunoreactive terminals in the monkey DLPFC form asymmetric synapses (Melchitzky et al. 1999), a morphological feature associated with excitatory terminals. Thus, refinements in the MD projections to the DLPFC during development may contribute to the maturational changes in parvalbumin varicosities shown in Figure 5–3, although direct investigations of these afferents during development remain to be conducted.

In the context of schizophrenia, potential developmental changes in projections from the MD are of interest given the evidence for disease-related disturbances in these afferents. As discussed earlier (see Figure 5–3D), the density of parvalbumin-positive varicosities is reduced selectively in the middle cortical layers (3b–4) in schizophrenia and is unchanged in the superficial layers (2–3a) of the DLPFC (Lewis et al. 2001). These data may be consistent with either the reported reduction in parvalbumin expression in GABA neurons in the middle cortical layers of subjects with schizophrenia (Hashimoto et al. 2003) or a decrease in the number of parvalbumin-containing axon terminals from the MD. Consistent with the latter interpretation, some but not all, studies have reported a reduced number of neurons in the MD in subjects with schizophrenia (Harrison and Lewis 2003).

Another afferent system to the DLPFC of particular relevance to working memory is the dopamine projection from the mesencephalon. A substantial set of findings indicates that the proper level of dopamine activity in the DLPFC is essential for normal working memory function (Goldman-Rakic 1998); innervation of monkey DLPFC also undergoes substantial changes during postnatal development (Goldman-Rakic and Brown 1982; Lewis and Harris 1991; Lidow et al. 1991). These afferents to the primate DLPFC form symmetric contacts with dendritic spines and shafts of pyramidal neurons (Goldman-Rakic et al. 1989; Smiley et al. 1992), as well as with the dendrites of local circuit neurons (Smiley and Goldman-Rakic 1993) that contain GABA (Sesack et al. 1995b). In addition, among GABA neurons in the monkey DLPFC, the dendrites of parvalbumin-containing cells in the middle cortical layers receive dopamine synaptic input (Gainetdinov et al. 1999), whereas the calretinin-containing class of GABA neurons in the superficial layers does not (Sesack et al. 1995a). Consequently, the maturational changes in the dopamine innervation of DLPFC layer 3 are of particular interest.

As summarized in Figure 5–4A, the density of varicosities (possible sites of synaptic specializations or neurotransmitter release) on dopamine axons (as suggested by immunoreactivity for tyrosine hydroxylase, a selective marker of dopamine axons in the cortex) in layer 3 of monkey DLPFC increases during the first few postnatal months (Rosenberg and Lewis 1995), parallel to the increase in densities of pyramidal neuron dendritic spines and parvalbumin-immunoreactive chandelier neuron axon cartridges. After a plateau period, dopamine varicosities undergo a second marked increase in density to reach peak values at age 2–3 years. The number of dopamine varicosities then rapidly declines to relatively stable adult levels by age 5 years. This second rise in the density of dopamine varicosities appears to begin before the decline in the densities of pyramidal neuron dendritic spines and parvalbumin-immunoreactive cartridges in layer 3 and to persist until the adult levels of these markers of excitatory and inhibitory inputs are achieved.

These patterns suggest that the neuromodulatory effects of dopamine may influence the adolescent refinement of excitatory and inhibitory inputs to layer 3 pyramidal neurons. In contrast, dopamine axons in other locations, such as layer 6, showed little evidence of refinements during the postnatal period (Rosenberg and Lewis 1995).

A large body of both preclinical and clinical literature supports the hypothesis that schizophrenia is associated with a functional deficit in the dopamine innervation of the DLPFC and that this disturbance contributes to the impairments in prefrontal-mediated cognitive processes in the illness (Goldman-Rakic 1999). Consideration of these observations in the context of the development of dopamine afferents is limited by the few studies that have examined the same measure in both monkeys and humans. Investigations of tyrosine hydroxylase–positive axon terminals reported a decrease in the dopamine innervation density

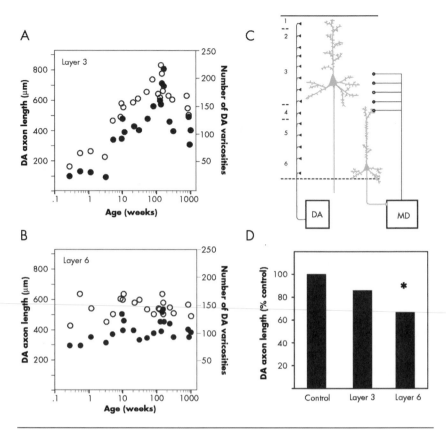

Figure 5–4. Development of dopaminergic axons and their alterations in schizophrenia are lamina-specific in the dorsolateral prefrontal cortex (DLPFC).

Panel A: Both the total axon length *(open circles)* and the number of varicosities *(filled circles)* immunoreactive for tyrosine hydroxylase, the rate-limiting enzyme in dopamine (DA) synthesis, change significantly in layer 3 during postnatal development in monkeys (adapted from Rosenberg and Lewis 1995). **Panel B:** Similar measures in layer 6 do not show marked developmental alterations. **Panel C:** The laminar specificity of developmental changes in DA innervation suggest differential modulation of particular elements of prefrontal circuitry. These include the pyramidal cells of layer 3, which form connections with both local and remote cortical areas, and those of layer 6, which are the source of descending, corticothalamic projections to the mediodorsal nucleus (MD). Cortical layers are indicated by *arabic numerals* at the left of the figure. **Panel D:** Postmortem studies show that the density of dopaminergic axons is reduced in these layers in schizophrenia; however, these changes reached significance (indicated by *asterisk*) only in layer 6 (adapted from Akil et al. 1999).

of the DLPFC of subjects with schizophrenia (Akil et al. 1999), but the statistically significant changes were restricted to layer 6 and were not found in layer 3, where the marked changes in dopamine innervation density occur during adolescence (Figure 5–4D). This difference in the laminar specificity of prominent developmental changes and significant postmortem observations in the dopamine system in schizophrenia presents a striking contrast to the cortical cell populations described in the preceding sections. These findings suggest that the functional deficit in DLPFC dopamine in schizophrenia does not represent an alteration in developmental trajectory of this neurotransmitter system and may instead reflect a disturbance that arises after this circuitry has matured.

Conclusion

The acquisition of mature levels of performance for cognitive processes involving executive control, such as working memory, appears to be delayed until early adulthood in monkeys and humans. These processes depend on the synchronized activity of neural networks in the DLPFC. In vivo electrophysiology, tract tracing, and lesion studies suggest that reciprocal excitatory connections among pyramidal cells, inhibitory regulation by fast-spiking (i.e., parvalbumin-containing) GABA neurons, and subcortical inputs from the MD thalamus and dopamine-containing cells are essential elements of these neural networks. The studies reviewed in this chapter indicate that each of these neural elements undergoes refinements during a protracted period of postnatal development that parallels the time course of maturation of working memory performance in primates. Most, but not all, of these neural elements are altered in schizophrenia, suggesting that the deficits in working memory in this illness may be the result of disruptions in the developmental trajectories of these neural elements. These temporal correlations may explain how various environmental factors (e.g., labor and delivery complications, urban place of rearing, and marijuana use during adolescence) are all associated with increased risk for the appearance of schizophrenia later in life.

References

Akil M, Pierri JN, Whitehead RE, et al: Lamina-specific alteration in the dopamine innervation of the prefrontal cortex in schizophrenic subjects. Am J Psychiatry 156:1580–1589, 1999

Alexander GE, Goldman PS: Functional development of the dorsolateral prefrontal cortex: an analysis utilizing reversible cryogenic depression. Brain Res 143:233–249, 1978

Anderson SA, Classey JD, Condé F, et al: Synchronous development of pyramidal neuron dendritic spines and parvalbumin-immunoreactive chandelier neuron axon terminals in layer III of monkey prefrontal cortex. Neuroscience 67:7–22, 1995

Andreasen NC, Rezai R, Alliger R, et al: Hypofrontality in neuroleptic-naive patients and in patients with chronic schizophrenia: assessment with xenon 133 single-photon emission computed tomography and the Tower of London. Arch Gen Psychiatry 49:943–958, 1992

Barch DM, Sheline YI, Csernansky JG, et al: Working memory and prefrontal cortex dysfunction: specificity to schizophrenia compared with major depression. Biol Psychiatry 53:376–384, 2003

Botvinick MM, Braver TS, Barch DM, et al: Conflict monitoring and cognitive control. Psychol Rev 108:624–652, 2001

Bourgeois J-P, Goldman-Rakic PS, Rakic P: Synaptogenesis in the prefrontal cortex of rhesus monkeys. Cereb Cortex 4:78–96, 1994

Buchsbaum M: The frontal lobes, basal ganglia and temporal lobes as sites for schizophrenia. Schizophr Bull 16:379–389, 1990

Callicott JH, Tallent K, Bertolino A, et al: fMRI brain mapping in psychiatry. Neuropsychopharmacology 18:186–196, 1998

Callicott JH, Mattay VS, Bertolino A, et al: Physiological characteristics of capacity constraints in working memory as revealed by functional MRI. Cereb Cortex 9:20–26, 1999

Callicott JH, Bertolino A, Mattay VS, et al: Physiological dysfunction of the dorsolateral prefrontal cortex in schizophrenia revisited. Cereb Cortex 10:1078–1092, 2000

Carter CS, Robertson L, Chaderjian M, et al: Attentional asymmetry in schizophrenia: controlled and automatic processes. Biol Psychiatry 31:909–918, 1992

Carter CS, Robertson L, Nordhal TE, et al: Spatial working memory deficits and their relationship to negative symptoms in unmedicated schizophrenic patients. Biol Psychiatry 40:930–932, 1996

Carter CS, Perlstein W, Ganguli R, et al: Functional hypofrontality and working memory dysfunction in schizophrenia. Am J Psychiatry 155:1285–1287, 1998

Carter CS, Botvinick M, Cohen JD: The contribution of the anterior cingulate cortex to executive processes in cognition. Rev Neurosci 10:49–57, 1999

Celio MR: Parvalbumin as a marker for fast firing neurons. Neurosci Lett 18:332, 1984

Cobb SR, Buhl EH, Halasy K, et al: Synchronization of neuronal activity in hippocampus by individual GABAergic interneurons. Nature 378:75–78, 1995

Cohen JD, Botvinick M, Carter CS: Anterior cingulate and prefrontal cortex: who's in control. Nat Neurosci 3:421–423, 2002

Condé F, Lund JS, Jacobowitz DM, et al: Local circuit neurons immunoreactive for calretinin, calbindin D-28k, or parvalbumin in monkey prefrontal cortex: distribution and morphology. J Comp Neurol 341:95–116, 1994

Cornblatt BA, Lenzenweger MF, Erlenmeyer-Kimling L: The Continuous Performance Test, Identical Pairs Version, II: contrasting attention profiles in schizophrenic and depressed patients. Psychiatry Res 29:65–85, 1989

Cosway R, Byrne M, Clafferty R, et al: Neuropsychological change in young people at high risk for schizophrenia: results from the first two neuropsychological assessments of the Edinburgh High Risk Study. Psychol Med 30:1111–1121, 2000

Cruz DA, Eggan SM, Lewis DA: Postnatal development of pre- and post-synaptic GABA markers at chandelier cell inputs to pyramidal neurons in monkey prefrontal cortex. J Comp Neurol 465:385–400, 2003

DeFelipe J, Farinas I: The pyramidal neuron of the cerebral cortex: morphological and chemical characteristics of the synaptic inputs. Prog Neurobiol 39:563–607, 1992

DeFelipe J, Jones EG: Parvalbumin immunoreactivity reveals layer IV of monkey cerebral cortex as a mosaic of microzones of thalamic afferent terminations. Brain Res 562:39–47, 1991

DeFelipe J, Hendry SHC, Jones EG: Visualization of chandelier cell axons by parvalbumin immunoreactivity in monkey cerebral cortex. Proc Natl Acad Sci U S A 86:2093–2097, 1989

Diamond A: Normal development of prefrontal cortex from birth to young adulthood: cognitive functions, anatomy and biochemistry, in Principles of Frontal Lobe Function. Edited by Knight SA. London, Oxford University Press, 2002, pp 466–503

Egan MF, Goldberg TE, Gscheidle T, et al: Relative risk for cognitive impairments in siblings of patients with schizophrenia. Biol Psychiatry 50:98–107, 2001

Elvevåg B, Goldberg TE: Cognitive impairment in schizophrenia is the core of the disorder. Crit Rev Neurobiol 14:1–21, 2000

Erickson SL, Lewis DA: Postnatal development of parvalbumin- and GABA transporter-immunoreactive axon terminals in monkey prefrontal cortex. J Comp Neurol 448:186–202, 2002

Erickson SL, Lewis DA: Cortical connections of the lateral mediodorsal nucleus in cynomolgus monkeys. J Comp Neurol (in press)

Fritschy J-M, Paysan J, Enna A, et al: Switch in the expression of rat GABAA-receptor subtypes during postnatal development: an immunohistochemical study. J Neurosci 14:5302–5324, 1994

Gainetdinov RR, Wetsel WC, Jones SR, et al: Role of serotonin in the paradoxical calming effect of psychostimulants on hyperactivity. Science 283:397–401, 1999

Garey LJ, Ong WY, Patel TS, et al: Reduced dendritic spine density on cerebral cortical pyramidal neurons in schizophrenia. J Neurol Neurosurg Psychiatry 65:446–453, 1998

Giguere M, Goldman-Rakic PS: Mediodorsal nucleus: areal, laminar, and tangential distribution of afferents and efferents in the frontal lobe of rhesus monkeys. J Comp Neurol 277:195–213, 1988

Gilbert CD, Wiesel TN: Columnar specificity of intrinsic horizontal and corticocortical connections in cat visual cortex. J Neurosci 9:2432–2442, 1989

Glantz LA, Lewis DA: Decreased dendritic spine density on prefrontal cortical pyramidal neurons in schizophrenia. Arch Gen Psychiatry 57:65–73, 2000

Gold JM, Carpenter C, Randolph C, et al: Auditory working memory and Wisconsin Card Sorting Test performance in schizophrenia. Arch Gen Psychiatry 54:159–165, 1997

Goldman-Rakic PS: Circuitry of primate prefrontal cortex and regulation of behavior by representational memory, in Handbook of Physiology, Vol 5. Edited by Plum F, Mountcastle V. Bethesda, MD, American Physiological Society, 1987, pp 373–417

Goldman-Rakic PS: Cellular basis of working memory. Neuron 14:477–485, 1995

Goldman-Rakic PS: The cortical dopamine system: role in memory and cognition, in Catecholamines: Bridging Basic Science With Clinical Medicine. Edited by Goldstein DS, Eisenhofer G, McCarty R. San Diego, CA, Academic Press, 1998, pp 707–711

Goldman-Rakic PS: The physiology approach: functional architecture of working memory and disordered cognition in schizophrenia. Biol Psychiatry 46:650–661, 1999

Goldman-Rakic PS, Brown RM: Postnatal development of monoamine content and synthesis in the cerebral cortex of rhesus monkeys. Dev Brain Res 4:339–349, 1982

Goldman-Rakic PS, Leranth C, Williams SM, et al: Dopamine synaptic complex with pyramidal neurons in primate cerebral cortex. Proc Natl Acad Sci U S A 86:9015–9019, 1989

Gottesman II: Schizophrenia Genesis: The Origins of Madness. New York, WH Freeman, 1991

Gottesman II, Bertelsen A: Confirming unexpressed genotypes for schizophrenia: risks in the offspring of Fischers's Danish identical and fraternal discordant twins. Arch Gen Psychiatry 46:867–872, 1989

Green MF: What are the functional consequences of neurocognitive deficits in schizophrenia? Am J Psychiatry 153:321–330, 1996

Green MF: Schizophrenia From a Neurocognitive Perspective: Probing the Impenetrable Darkness. Boston, MA, Allyn & Bacon, 1998

Gur RC, Gur RE: Hypofrontality in schizophrenia: RIP. Lancet 345:1383–1384, 1995

Harrison PJ, Lewis DA: Neuropathology in schizophrenia, in Schizophrenia, 2nd Edition. Edited by Hirsch S, Weinberger DR. Oxford, UK, Blackwell Science, 2003, pp 310–325

Harvey PD, Howanitz E, Parrella M, et al: Symptoms, cognitive functioning, and adaptive skills in geriatric patients with lifelong schizophrenia: a comparison across treatment sites. Am J Psychiatry 155:1080–1086, 1998

Hashimoto T, Volk DW, Eggan SM, et al: Gene expression deficits in a subclass of GABA neurons in the prefrontal cortex of subjects with schizophrenia. J Neurosci 23:6315–6326, 2003

Hirsch JA, Gilbert CD: Synaptic physiology of horizontal connections in the cat's visual cortex. J Neurosci 11:1800–1809, 1991

Ingraham LJ, Kety SS: Adoption studies of schizophrenia. Am J Med Genet 97:18–22, 2000

Jones EG, Hendry SHC: Basket cells, in Cerebral Cortex, Vol 1: Cellular Components of the Cerebral Cortex. Edited by Jones EG, Peters A. New York, Plenum, 1984, pp 309–336

Jones EG, Hendry SHC: Differential calcium binding protein immunoreactivity distinguishes classes of relay neurons in monkey thalamic nuclei. Eur J Neurosci 1:222–246, 1989

Keefe RSE, Roitman SEL, Harvey PD, et al: A pen-and-paper human analogue of a monkey prefrontal cortex activation task: spatial working memory in patients with schizophrenia. Schizophr Res 17:25–33, 1995

Kety SS, Rosenthal D, Wender PH, et al: Mental illness in the biological and adoptive families of adopted schizophrenics. Am J Psychiatry 128:82–86, 1971

Klausberger T, Magill PJ, Marton LF, et al: Brain-state- and cell-type specific firing of hippocampal interneurons in vivo. Nature 421:844–848, 2003

Kritzer MF, Goldman-Rakic PS: Intrinsic circuit organization of the major layers and sublayers of the dorsolateral prefrontal cortex in the rhesus monkey. J Comp Neurol 359:131–143, 1995

Kuroda M, Murakami K, Oda S, et al: Direct synaptic connections between thalamocortical axon terminals from the mediodorsal thalamic nucleus (MD) and corticothalamic neurons to MD in the prefrontal cortex. Brain Res 612:339–344, 1993

Lavoie AM, Tingey JJ, Harrison NL, et al: Activation and deactivation rates of recombinant $GABA_A$ receptor channels are dependent on α-subunit isoform. Biophys J 73:2518–2526, 1997

Levitt JB, Lewis DA, Yoshioka T, et al: Topography of pyramidal neuron intrinsic connections in macaque monkey prefrontal cortex (areas 9 and 46). J Comp Neurol 338:360–376, 1993

Lewis DA: Development of the primate prefrontal cortex, in Neurodevelopment and Adult Psychopathology. Edited by Keshavan MS, Murray RM. Cambridge, England, Cambridge University Press, 1997, pp 12–30

Lewis DA, Anderson SA: The functional architecture of the prefrontal cortex and schizophrenia. Psychol Med 25:887–894, 1995

Lewis DA, Gonzalez-Burgos G: Intrinsic excitatory connections in the prefrontal cortex and the pathophysiology of schizophrenia. Brain Res Bull 52:309–317, 2000

Lewis DA, Harris HW: Differential laminar distribution of tyrosine hydroxylase-immunoreactive axons in infant and adult monkey prefrontal cortex. Neurosci Lett 125:151–154, 1991

Lewis DA, Levitt P: Schizophrenia as a disorder of neurodevelopment. Annu Rev Neurosci 25:409–432, 2002

Lewis DA, Lieberman JA: Catching up on schizophrenia: natural history and neurobiology. Neuron 28:325–334, 2000

Lewis DA, Lund JS: Heterogeneity of chandelier neurons in monkey neocortex: corticotropin-releasing factor and parvalbumin immunoreactive populations. J Comp Neurol 293:599–615, 1990

Lewis DA, Cruz DA, Melchitzky DS, et al: Lamina-specific deficits in parvalbumin-immunoreactive varicosities in the prefrontal cortex of subjects with schizophrenia: evidence for fewer projections from the thalamus. Am J Psychiatry 158:1411–1422, 2001

Lewis DA, Melchitzky DS, Burgos GG: Specificity in the functional architecture of primate prefrontal cortex. J Neurocytol 31:265–276, 2002

Lidow MS, Goldman-Rakic PS, Rakic P: Synchronized overproduction of neurotransmitter receptors in diverse regions of the primate cerebral cortex. Proc Natl Acad Sci U S A 88:10218–10221, 1991

Loup F, Weinmann O, Yonekawa Y, et al: A highly sensitive immunofluorescence procedure for analyzing the subcellular distribution of $GABA_A$ receptor subunits in the human brain. J Histochem Cytochem 46:1129–1139, 1998

Lund JS, Lewis DA: Local circuit neurons of developing and mature macaque prefrontal cortex: Golgi and immunocytochemical characteristics. J Comp Neurol 328:282–312, 1993

Manoach DS, Press DZ, Thangaraj V, et al: Schizophrenic subjects activate dorsolateral prefrontal cortex during a working memory task, as measured by fMRI. Biol Psychiatry 45:1128–1137, 1999

McFarland NR, Haber SN: Thalamic relay nuclei of the basal ganglia form both reciprocal and nonreciprocal cortical connections, linking multiple frontal cortical areas. J Neurosci 22:8117–8132, 2002

Melchitzky DS, Sesack SR, Lewis DA: Parvalbumin-immunoreactive axon terminals in macaque monkey and human prefrontal cortex: laminar, regional and target specificity of Type I and Type II synapses. J Comp Neurol 408:11–22, 1999

Mirsky AF: Neuropsychological bases of schizophrenia. Annu Rev Psychol 20:321–348, 1969

Neuchterlein KH, Dawson ME: Information processing and attentional functioning in the developmental course of schizophrenia disorders. Schizophr Bull 10:160–203, 1984

Park S, Holzman PS: Schizophrenics show spatial working memory deficits. Arch Gen Psychiatry 49:975–982, 1992

Peters A: Chandelier cells, in Cerebral Cortex, Vol 1: Cellular Components of the Cerebral Cortex. Edited by Jones EG, Peters A. New York, Plenum, 1984, pp 361–380

Pierri JN, Chaudry AS, Woo T-U, et al: Alterations in chandelier neuron axon terminals in the prefrontal cortex of schizophrenic subjects. Am J Psychiatry 156:1709–1719, 1999

Posner MI, Di Girolamo GJ: Executive attention: conflict, target detection, and cognitive control, in The Attentive Brain. Edited by Parasuraman R. Cambridge, MA, MIT Press, 1998, pp 401–423

Pucak ML, Levitt JB, Lund JS, et al: Patterns of intrinsic and associational circuitry in monkey prefrontal cortex. J Comp Neurol 376:614–630, 1996

Rosenberg DR, Lewis DA: Postnatal maturation of the dopaminergic innervation of monkey prefrontal and motor cortices: a tyrosine hydroxylase immunohistochemical analysis. J Comp Neurol 358:383–400, 1995

Sesack SR, Bressler CN, Lewis DA: Ultrastructural associations between dopamine terminals and local circuit neurons in the monkey prefrontal cortex: a study of calretinin-immunoreactive cells. Neurosci Lett 200:9–12, 1995a

Sesack SR, Snyder CL, Lewis DA: Axon terminals immunolabeled for dopamine or tyrosine hydroxylase synapse on GABA-immunoreactive dendrites in rat and monkey cortex. J Comp Neurol 363 264–280, 1995b

Shallice T: From Neuropsychology to Mental Structure. Cambridge, UK, Cambridge University Press, 1988

Smiley JF, Goldman-Rakic PS: Heterogeneous targets of dopamine synapses in monkey prefrontal cortex demonstrated by serial section electron microscopy: a laminar analysis using the silver-enhanced diaminobenzidine sulfide (SEDS) immunolabeling technique. Cereb Cortex 3:223–238, 1993

Smiley JF, Williams SM, Szigeti K, et al: Light and electron microscopic characterization of dopamine-immunoreactive axons in human cerebral cortex. J Comp Neurol 321:325–335, 1992

Smith EE, Jonides J: Storage and executive processes in the frontal lobes. Science 283:1657–1661, 1999

Taylor SF: Cerebral blood flow activation and functional lesions in schizophrenia. Schizophr Res 19:129–140, 1996

Tsuang MT, Stone WS, Faraone SV: Genes, environment and schizophrenia. Br J Psychiatry 40S:18–24, 2001

Tucker TR, Katz LC: Recruitment of local inhibitory networks by horizontal connections in layer 2/3 of ferret visual cortex. J Neurophysiol 89:501–512, 2003

Volk DW, Austin MC, Pierri JN, et al: Decreased GAD_{67} mRNA expression in a subset of prefrontal cortical GABA neurons in subjects with schizophrenia. Arch Gen Psychiatry 57:237–245, 2000

Volk DW, Austin MC, Pierri JN, et al: GABA transporter-1 mRNA in the prefrontal cortex in schizophrenia: decreased expression in a subset of neurons. Am J Psychiatry 158:256–265, 2001

Volk DW, Pierri JN, Fritschy J-M, et al: Reciprocal alterations in pre- and postsynaptic inhibitory markers at chandelier cell inputs to pyramidal neurons in schizophrenia. Cereb Cortex 12:1063–1070, 2002

Weinberger DR, Berman KF, Zec RF: Physiologic dysfunction of dorsolateral prefrontal cortex in schizophrenia, I: regional cerebral blood flow evidence. Arch Gen Psychiatry 43:114–124, 1986

Weinberger DR, Berman KF, Illowsky BP: Physiological dysfunction of dorsolateral prefrontal cortex in schizophrenia, III: a new cohort and evidence for a monoaminergic mechanism. Arch Gen Psychiatry 45:609–615, 1988

Weinberger DR, Egan MF, Bertolino A, et al: Prefrontal neurons and the genetics of schizophrenia. Biol Psychiatry 50:825–844, 2001

White EL: Cortical Circuits. Boston, MA, Birkhauser, 1989, pp 32–34

Woo T-U, Pucak ML, Kye CH, et al: Peripubertal refinement of the intrinsic and associational circuitry in monkey prefrontal cortex. Neuroscience 80:1149–1158, 1997

Woo T-U, Whitehead RE, Melchitzky DS, et al: A subclass of prefrontal gamma-aminobutyric acid axon terminals are selectively altered in schizophrenia. Proc Natl Acad Sci U S A 95:5341–5346, 1998

Index

Page numbers printed in **boldface** *type refer to tables or figures.*

Autism *(continued)*
　　face recognition and, 46–47,
　　　48–49, 49–50
Autoimmune mechanisms, in
　　Tourette's syndrome,
　　116, 130
Axon initial segment (AIS),
　　of pyramidal neurons,
　　151–152

Basal ganglia
　　excitatory corticofugal
　　　　projections to, tics and, 117
　　subcortical nuclei of, 117, **118**
　　in Tourette's syndrome,
　　　126–127
Blood pressure, maternal
　　behavior related to, 19–20
Bowlby's attachment theory, 2–4
Brain.
　　See also specific regions of brain
　　in learning
　　　experience dependent, xvii
　　　experience expectant, xvii
　　recent research about, xi–xiv

Cartridges, of dorsolateral
　　prefrontal cortex neurons,
　　155–156, **155,** 159
Caudate, 117, **118**
Cerebral pathology,
　　Tourette's syndrome and, 128
Cerebral volumes,
　　in Tourette's syndrome, 130
Chandelier neurons,
　　of dorsolateral prefrontal
　　cortex, **147,** 153, 154–157,
　　155, 159
Children
　　autistic, face recognition in,
　　　46–47, **48–49,** 49–50

reading disability in
　　interventions for, 94–95,
　　　96–98, 99–102
　　neuroimaging studies of,
　　　83, **84–86,** 87–91
　　recognition of inverted faces
　　　by, 40
Cognitive deficits
　　reading disability and, 70–72
　　in schizophrenia, 144–146
Cognitive tasks
　　fMRI and, 31
　　reading disability in adults,
　　　74–80
Configural information,
　　face processing and, 40–41
CONLERN mechanism, 54, 58
CONSPEC mechanism, 50–51, 58
Corpus callosum,
　　in Tourette's syndrome, 130
Cortical recruitment, increased,
　　in reading disorder, 90–91
Cortical specialization,
　　face processing and, 58
Corticosterone, maternal-infant
　　separation and, 15
Cortico-striato-thalamo-cortical
　　circuits
　　anatomical features of, 117, **118**
　　in Tourette's syndrome,
　　　124–125
Corticotropin, maternal-infant
　　separation and, 15
Critical periods, for
　　developmental learning, xvii
Cytogenetic abnormalities, in
　　Tourette's syndrome, 114

Developmental learning
　　characteristics of, xvii–xix,
　　　xviii

Infants
  face processing in, 36–37, **38,** 39
    CONSPEC mechanism and,
      50–51, 58
    experience and, 56–57
    face discrimination and,
      33–34
    facial expression and
      emotion processing
      and, 42–43
    right hemisphere and, 54–55
    sensory hypothesis of,
      52–54, **53**
    visual preferences and,
      51–52
  isolation call associated with
    separation from mother,
    11–14
  orientation to mother, 8–9
  premature, maternal
    separation and, 11
  recognition and preference for
    own mother, learning of,
    6–7
  speech processing and risk for
    reading disorder in, 91–92
Inhibitory interneurons, of
    dorsolateral prefrontal
    cortex, postnatal
    development of, 153–157, **155**
Insular cortex, left, reading
    disability and, 73, 81
Interneurons, of dorsolateral
    prefrontal cortex, 146, **147**
  postnatal development of, 148,
    149, 150–153
Inverted faces, recognition of,
    35–36, 40
Ischemia, perinatal, Tourette's
    syndrome and, 115
Isolation call, 11–14

Learning
  developmental
    characteristics of, xvii–xix,
      xviii
    mechanisms underlying,
      xix–xxi
  fetal, attachment and, 6
  olfactory, early, 7

Magnetic resonance imaging
    (MRI).
    See also Functional magnetic
      resonance imaging (fMRI)
    impact on field, xxiv–xxvi
Magnetoencephalography (MEG)
  in reading-disabled adults,
    73, **74–80,** 81–82
  in reading-disabled children,
    84, 88–89, 90, **97**
  usefulness of, 100–101
    during visual pseudoword
      task, 95, 99
Maternal behavior
  interaction with genetic
    predisposition, 18–20
  later regulatory interactions
    and, 22–23
  mental representations and,
    21–22
  separation from infant and,
    16–24
  transgenerational
    transmission of,
    17–18
Maternal-infant attachment.
    See Attachment
Matrisomes, **120,** 124
Medium spiny projection (MSP)
    neurons, in Tourette's
    syndrome, 119, **119, 120,** 121
  dysregulated firing of, 124

Startle reflex,
in Tourette's syndrome, 132
State-dependent regional
activations, in Tourette's
syndrome, 128
Still-face effect, 42
"The Strange Situation," 2
Stress diathesis model,
of Tourette's syndrome
pathogenesis, 115–116
Stress-hyporesponsive period,
14–16
Striatum, 117, **118**
in Tourette's syndrome, 127
dopaminergic innervation
of, 126
Striosomes, **118, 120,** 121
Structural imaging studies,
in Tourette's syndrome,
129–130
Substantia nigra, 117, **118**
Subthalamic nucleus (STN),
117, **118**
in Tourette's syndrome, **120,**
124–125, 126
Superior temporal gyrus, left,
reading disability and,
73, 87
Supramarginal gyrus, left,
reading disability and, 73
Sydenham's chorea, 116, 130

Task difficulty,
dorsolateral prefrontal cortex
activity correlated with, 145
Temporal cortex
face recognition and, 45
left posterior regions of,
reading disability and, 73
Temporal gyrus,
face recognition and, 46–47

Thalamus, mediodorsal nucleus
of, parvalbumin and, 157–158
Tic disorders.
See Tourette's syndrome
Tonically active neurons (TANs),
in Tourette's syndrome,
121–123
Tourette's syndrome, xxiii,
111–135
comorbidity of, 113
environmental factors in,
115–116
epidemiology and genetics of,
113–116
fMRI studies of, 129
future research directions for,
133–135
neural substrates of habit
formation and tics and,
116–117, **118–120,** 119–125
neuroimaging of, adults with,
127, 129, 130
neuroimmunological findings
in, 130–131
neuropathological studies of,
125–126
neurophysiological studies of,
131–132
neuropsychological findings
in, 131
neurosurgical interventions
for, 128
secondary to cerebral
malignancies or infarction,
128
structural imaging studies of,
129–130
symptoms and natural history
of, 111–113
tic facilitators in, **120**
tic initiators in, **119**